Disclaimer

This e-book has been written for information purposes only. Every effort has been made to make this e-book as complete and accurate as possible. However, there may be mistakes in typography or content. Also, this e-book provides information only up to the publishing date. Therefore, this e-book should be used as a guide - not as the ultimate source.

The purpose of this e-book is to educate. The author and the publisher do not warrant that the information contained in this e- book is fully complete and shall not be responsible for any errors or omissions. The author and publisher shall have neither liability nor responsibility to any person or entity with respect to any loss or damage caused or alleged to be caused directly or indirectly by this e-book.

Introduction

When we start to grow older, several changes take place in our body - and these changes often work as a chain reaction.

One change will lead to another. These changes take place in both men and women and contribute to the ageing process.

Men usually notice these changes first when they begin to experience lower levels of the testosterone hormone.

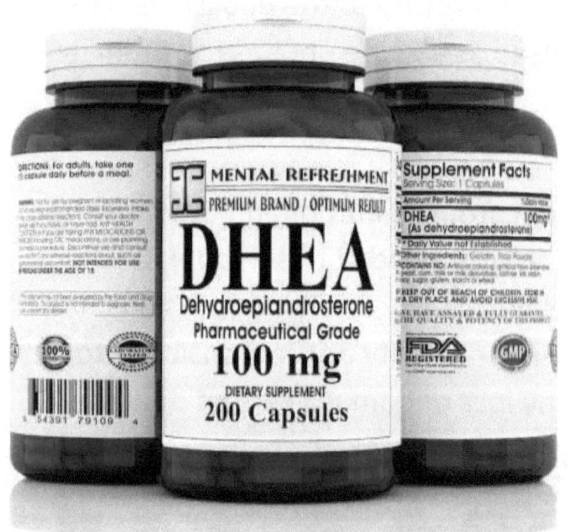

Their sex drive is off, they don't feel the same physically and emotionally and they may begin to see baldness occur.

Women lose estrogen, but they also lose DHEA.

This hormone is found in the adrenals and is doled out to different hormones within the body.

DHEA works as a control tower to help other hormones do what they're supposed to do.

In a small, six-week study, researchers from the National Institute of Mental Health found that treatment with DHEA supplements helped relieve mild to moderate depression that occurs in some middle-aged people. DHEA may also be effective for improving aging skin in the elderly.

Without enough DHEA, our metabolism becomes erratic, and we end up not being able to burn fat the way you used to, which in turn leads to weight gain.

DHEA can keep ageing at a slower rate and having enough of this hormone helps stabilise muscles and fight against bone density loss. It gives energy and improves sex drive.

With the lessening of certain hormones, our body just simply doesn't function the way it should and the aging process kicks in.

As these levels of hormones drop, you lose the benefit that hormones give the body.

We must have testosterone and estrogen in our battle against ageing, but there's another hormone we need, too. As you get older, you begin to have lower levels of the human growth hormone (or HGH).

Not having enough HGH robs the body of energy and weakens muscles. Without enough of this hormone, the skin will sag and bag and wrinkles and lines multiply. We begin to develop bone and joint problems and can experience problems with our heart.

We must have the proper hormones in order to prevent inflammations and serious health risks associated with ageing. Taking hormones like HGH helps the skin hold on to its suppleness.

It prevents hair loss - and this hormone is also beneficial to the immune system. For men, HGH works to fight against erectile dysfunction. This hormone can increase energy and improve memory function.

Testosterone is needed for energy and slows the aging process. It's also needed in order to keep muscles strong. Estrogen hormones keep the memory strong, fights against heart attacks and adds to longevity. It also prevents aging of the skin. Without enough estrogen, both hair and skin can begin to thin.

Another hormone with beneficial anti-ageing properties is melatonin. This hormone has antioxidants that fight against aging. It protects against cell damage both inside and outside the body. Supplements containing these hormones can provide anti-ageing benefits for us, but always check with your doctor before taking any type of supplement.

Natural Anti-ageing Therapy

There are many painful steps you can take to look younger. One process - known as laser skin resurfacing - is both expensive and painful.

Laser resurfacing is a specialist procedure to remove the outer layers of the skin from your face, aimed at encouraging new skin to grow.

People generally opt for this laser procedure for cosmetic reasons. It may be able to remove wrinkles, scars and areas of discolouration, and tighten your skin. If you think there must be a better way that you can look younger at home, you would be correct.

You'll see a vast amount of anti-ageing products for sale both locally and through online stores. They're in massive demand, because even though there's no such thing as the fountain of youth, anti-ageing products come close to that description.

They work to prevent the **signs** of ageing as well as reverse the signs that have already crept up on you.

As with any product line, some natural anti-ageing therapies are going to be better than others. Health studies show anti-ageing therapies that are successful depend on what the product contains.

Therapies high in minerals and vitamins - all natural - are better for the skin.

Your skin is under attack as you go about your day, and even while you're sound asleep. While you're asleep, your skin is under attack by the processes that cause you to look older.

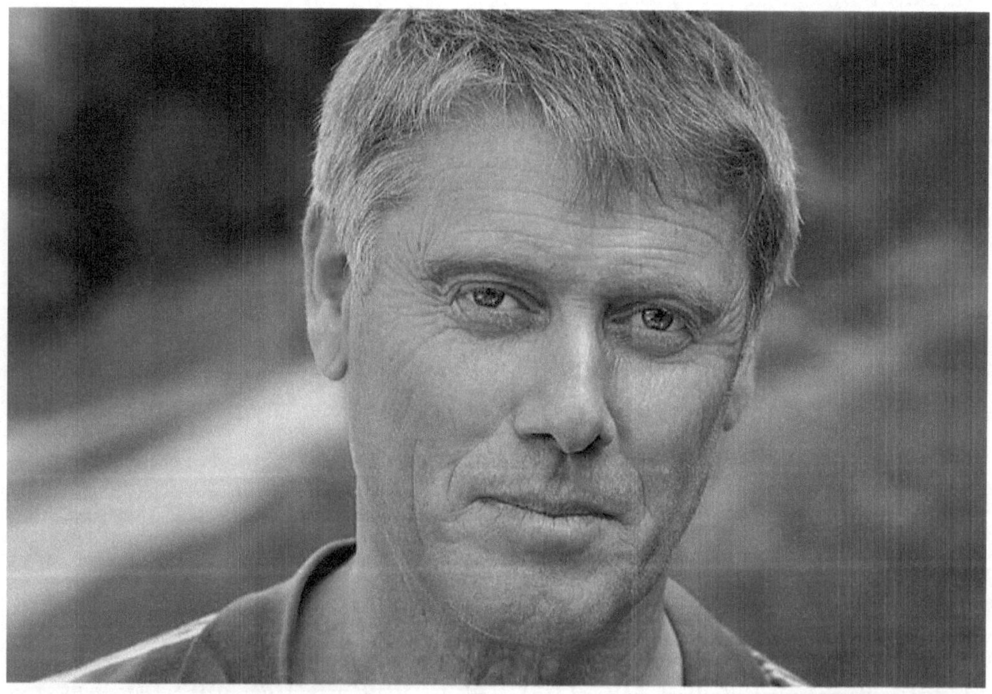

Lines are deepening, collagen is losing its tightness and age spots are developing. You might not see any of these changes outwardly for years. But having a consistent plan in place before you actually show signs of ageing will give you a jumpstart on great looking skin for your lifetime.

Even if your skin is already showing signs of ageing such as wrinkling, lines or dryness - you can still reverse the effects. You just need to start an anti-ageing routine right away. Protecting your skin from further damage will help you look younger.

Yes, we're forever told that whenever we're going to be out in the sun, use sunscreen, but the reality is, not just any sunscreen will do. You need an anti-ageing sunscreen. Many of these are SPF 15 and higher (the higher the better) and are made from organic ingredients, which are better for your skin.

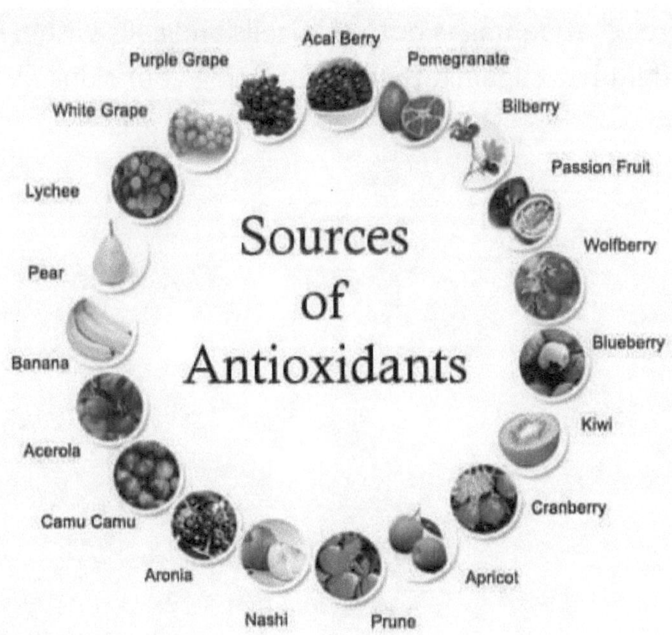

Look for anti-ageing solutions that specifically label themselves as antioxidant or as age reversing treatments. You might also see some solutions that offer antioxidants that release small increments of protection throughout the day.

When you clean your face, always clean with an anti-ageing cleanser, followed by an anti-ageing moisturiser to keep your skin hydrated. Because free radicals are what damages both skin cells and cells within the body, you want to fight back against them, protecting your skin from further damage.

What Goes into Anti-ageing creams?

Moisturising pure and simple can indeed improve the appearance of your skin because it temporarily plumps up the skin and makes lines and wrinkles less visible.

Leave a raisin or sultana in water overnight and that wrinkled dried fruit will plump up!

Moisturisers come in many guises such as lotions, creams, gels and serums made of water, oils and other ingredients, such as proteins, waxes, glycerine, lactate and urea.

Glycerine (also known as glycerol) is a naturally occurring alcohol compound found in all animal, plant, and human tissues, including the skin and blood. Glycerine used in cosmetics can be obtained from natural sources such as soybeans, cane, or corn syrup sugar or manufactured synthetically.

Lactate is an organic molecule produced by most tissues in the human body, with the highest production found in muscle

Urea (also known as carbamide) is a waste product of many living organisms and is the major organic component of human urine. This is because it is at the end of chain of reactions which break down the amino acids that make up proteins.

Wrinkle creams often are moisturisers that contain active ingredients that provide additional benefits intended to improve skin tone, texture, fine lines and wrinkles.

The effectiveness of these wrinkle creams depends in part on your skin type and the active ingredient or ingredients.

There are some common ingredients that may result in some improvement in our skins appearance and outlined below.

- **Retinoids.** This term is used for **vitamin A** compounds, such as retinol and retinoic acid. Used as a cream/gel to help repair sun-damaged skin and reduce fine lines and wrinkles.

- **Vitamin C (ascorbic acid).** Vitamin C is a potent antioxidant, which means it protects the skin from free radicals — unstable oxygen molecules that break down skin cells and cause wrinkles. Vitamin C may help protect skin from sun damage and reduce fine lines and wrinkles.

- **Hydroxy acids.** Alpha hydroxy acids (AHAs) include glycolic, citric and lactic acid. They are used to remove dead skill cells (exfoliate). Using an AHA product regularly prepares your skin to better absorb other products and stimulates the growth of smooth, evenly pigmented new skin.

- **Coenzyme Q10.** This ingredient may help reduce fine wrinkles around the eyes and protect the skin from sun damage.

- **Peptides.** These molecules occur naturally in living organisms. Certain peptides are able to stimulate collagen production and have been shown to improve skin texture and wrinkling.

- **Tea extracts.** Green, black and oolong tea contain compounds with antioxidant and anti-inflammatory properties. Wrinkle creams are most likely to use green tea extracts.
- **Grape seed extract.** In addition to its antioxidant and anti-inflammatory properties, grape seed extract promotes collagen production.
- **Niacinamide.** A potent antioxidant, this substance is related to vitamin B-3 (niacin). It helps reduce water loss in the skin and may improve skin elasticity.

An expensive moisturiser or famous brand anti-ageing lotion may not be any better than a lower cost product, it's not the fancy label or price tag that makes it work, it's the ingredients.

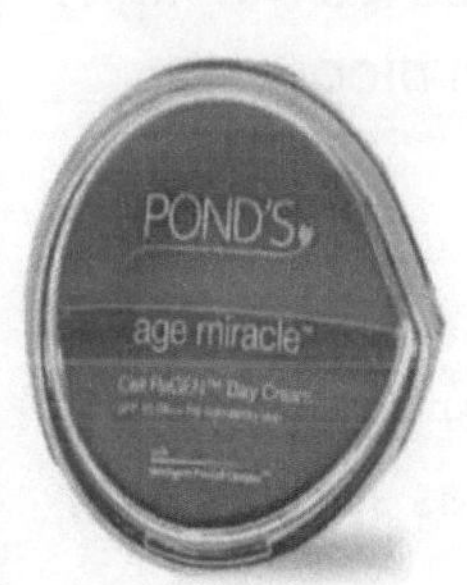

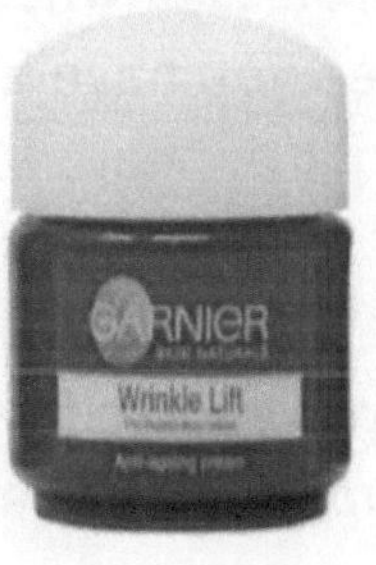

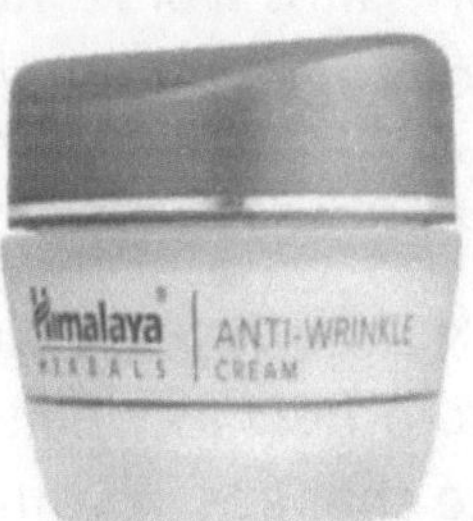

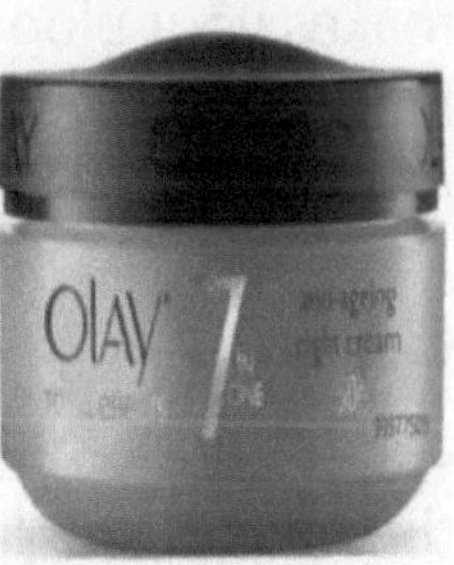

A basic moisturiser that makes no claims about anti-ageing doesn't necessarily mean it doesn't work as well as one that shouts about its anti-ageing properties – compare ingredients!

How Stress Steals Years Off Your Life

Stress does more than simply make you feel frazzled and worn out. It steals years off your life. You may not even realize that this is what's going on, but if you're dealing with stress, your body's ageing process is ticking along faster than you think.

High Blood Pressure

Whenever you get stressed, your body kicks into high gear and starts pumping out hormones as a reaction to that stress. As that happens, the hormones push your blood pressure to rise because it speeds up your heart rate.

High blood pressure causes narrowing of the arteries, which in turn makes your blood pressure worse. Regardless of what causes the high blood pressure, it does age you. But when you have high blood pressure due to stress, it also impacts your appearance.

You can start to look several years older than what you actually are - and it's noticeable to others as well as well yourself when you look in the mirror. You'll see changes in your appearance in areas such as your skin and in your face.

High blood pressure can cause saggy areas on your face as well as facial flushing. It also affects the way your blood pressure ages your mind. It speeds up the ageing process in your brain.

Your brain can't withstand chronically elevated high blood pressure without any negative side effects. Pressure in the veins from high blood pressure translates to pressure within the brain.

One study showed that a person who has high blood pressure can experience the same brain changes and brain ageing of someone nearly a decade older. That means that if someone's ageing process is sped up by stress, they're experiencing altered function and if it's not relieved, it can lead to subtle damage within the brain.

The longer it lasts, the more damage is done - and this damage can start as early as in your 20s. Whenever the stress is consistent, it causes fatigue because your blood isn't circulating as easily.

Your heart is working twice as hard. When you have high blood pressure, it increases your risks of what's commonly considered ageing diseases. Some of these medical conditions are kidney disease, heart failure, artery damage and stroke.

You can fight the effects of stress and slow or reverse the ageing process. The best way to do this is to understand that your blood pressure is something that needs to be checked regularly - even if you're young.

By keeping an eye on your blood pressure, you can bring it back down before it has a chance to cause damage. One way to track it is by having your doctor check it when you go in for a health checkup.

But you can also check your blood pressure at many pharmacies, or you can use machines at home. By getting into the habit of watching your blood pressure for any elevations, you can make the necessary changes.

Blood Sugar Spikes

Whenever you get stressed, your body goes into a fight or flight mode. It doesn't matter if it's a small stressor or a big stressor, the response that your body gives is the same.
You get a sudden burst of glucose in reaction to the stress.

While this response is helpful during a normal stress event - such as when you've had a scare and need to react quickly, the response is not helpful when you're dealing with the kind of stress that sticks around.

Your insulin levels will remain elevated the entire time you're under stress, and this is bad for your body. High levels of glucose in your bloodstream wreak havoc on your body because it can speed up the ageing process.

When you have extra sugar in your bloodstream, it starts to visually age your body. It does this outwardly by causing the appearance of dark circles beneath your eyes. It's also a contributing factor in skin blemishes.

Wrinkles can be a by-product of elevated glucose. One of the reasons for this is because whenever glucose is elevated due to stress, it dries out your skin. The elevated glucose, when a direct result of stress, ages your body because it causes dehydration and affects collagen production.

So, their skin ends up not looking as smooth and can be prone to splitting on the hands, elbows and heels of the feet. Studies show that people who live with stress and experience above normal blood glucose spikes end up looking older than people who manage their stress.

It also affects your body internally. People who experience elevated blood sugar spikes regularly can end up with similar health problems that both diabetics and the elderly experience.

It doesn't take an extremely high spike to cause ageing effects in the body, either. As little as twenty points above what's considered the normal range can have an effect.
When you experience blood sugar spikes, the elevated glucose keeps your body from healing the way it should.

This isn't just with things like cuts or sores or bruises, either. If you work out and you have blood glucose spikes caused by stress, your muscle recovery period will increase, and you'll find that your body recovers like someone who's much older.

The elevated glucose is preventing your muscles from snapping back the way that they normally would. Spikes in your blood sugar can cause you to feel mentally drained as well as physically fatigued, too.

Pain and Inflammation

Research has shown that whenever you're under stress it affects the ageing process by making you susceptible to pain as well as inflammation. Pain and inflammation are a direct result of the body reacting the stress that you're under.

It causes both short- and long-term responses in the body. In the short term, you might feel a stomach ache or develop muscle aches. But over time, you can develop conditions such as ulcers or chronic muscle pain or weakness due to the stress.

The answer to why this happens is found deep within the body - in the cells, to be exact. When you live your life as healthy as possible and you effectively deal with your stress, you don't experience pain or inflammation other than in normal circumstances.

Stress kills off what you need to keep you alive. When you're under stress, it causes the telomeres, found on the end of the chromosomes to shorten. As these cells shorten, you lose years off your life.

When you're stressed and it causes pain and inflammation, your cells begin to shorten faster and faster. Stress is literally speeding up your body's countdown clock. Over time, your cells lose the ability to divide and they die off.

The more stress you're under, the faster the process is. Studies found that people who live with stress are more likely to lose at least a decade and sometimes more of life. In these studies, it was found that the link between emotions strongly connected to the body's telomere cycle.

Another thing that stress does in the area of pain and inflammation is that it can make the body more susceptible to increased levels of pain and inflammation, and it can lower the threshold for developing conditions associated with ageing such as heart disease.

When you develop stress related inflammation, it speeds up your body's ageing process because of cytokines. These are secreted by the body whenever something health related is going on that needs to be addressed.

Normally, when a person is sick, these cytokines go to work to make you well again and then all is good. But when you're under stress, your body releases cytokines and they don't go away.

Instead, they stick around and start to create havoc. They create an inflammatory response within the body that doesn't go away. This is one way that people can develop chronic inflammatory health issues and it begins to take a toll on the body.

The result of this leads to what's known as oxidative damage. People who experience this then develop regenerative halting in their cells and tissues, which is part of accelerated ageing.

Immune System Deterioration

Your immune system is meant to protect you from foreign invaders. It's supposed to keep you safe from foreign invaders that you might pick up through your skin, or through breathing them.

It's supposed to protect you from bacteria and more. But when you deal with stress, it speeds up the ageing process and causes your immune system to deteriorate. That's because stress always suppresses the function of the immune system.

One way that it does this is by creating a shortage of the amount of white blood cells in the body. You need these cells to fight off both small and large infections. The minute your white blood cells decrease, your chances of getting sick go up.

When you get sick, your body is supposed to immediately send out the signal and rush healing cells throughout your body. Whatever the bacteria or virus is, your immune system is supposed to attack it and get whatever is making you sick out of there.

But stress hampers your immune system's ability to work because the stress hormone basically puts a leash on the system. It holds it back and prevents your system from working right.

A weakened immune system then begins to get overwhelmed, unable to keep up with the demands. T cell function naturally declines as a person gets older, but stress impacts the decline of T cell function in the immune system, regardless of your age.

Insomnia

Stress affects your health from head to toe, and it also affects your ability to get the amount of sleep that you need - which, of course, makes your health worse. When you're under stress, you lie awake and it's difficult to shut off your mind.

You can't relax and your body stays in a position of tenseness as well as wakefulness. Sometimes people with stress related insomnia find that they might fall asleep for a few minutes, but then they wake right back up.

They can't stay asleep. When this happens, the next day, they struggle to keep up with the physical and mental demands of their life. So they feel stressed about that, which only acerbates the stress and keeps the insomnia going.

Your body needs the rest and restoration that sleep provides. If it doesn't get it, several things begin to take place that speed up the ageing process. One of these things is cell changes.

When you have insomnia, the cells in your body begin to age. Studies show that people who suffer from insomnia have increased cell age and lose regenerative advances within the cells.

This damage and ageing cell reaction will show up in things like wrinkles, lines and bags on your face. The pigment beneath the eyes will begin to darken. Lines and grooves on the skin can deepen.

On the inside of your body, the cell damage and lack of regenerative supply speeds up health conditions and diseases that occur as a result of growing older. People who suffer with insomnia can experience a deficiency in growth hormone.

They'll experience fatigue and loss of muscle strength, both of which are associated with ageing but brought on by stress. And it doesn't take several months for insomnia to take a toll on the body. You can experience ageing changes in as little as one night of sleeplessness.

Mood Disorders

When you're under stress, it elevates the odds that a mood disorder is going to worsen. It doesn't matter if you've been doing fine lately. Stress changes everything. In many people, the stress that they encounter usually causes or adds to depression.

It's also known to increase anxiety. Studies have shown there's a direct link between mental health and stress. Stress causes an immediate change within the brain. When you encounter stress, the brain signals for certain chemicals to be released.

This is an attempt by the body to deal with the demands that stress is placing on your system. Your emotions are revved up and the brain is releasing these chemicals in an attempt to soothe them.

During this process, the production of stress hormones is also kicked up a notch. This is the hormone that's responsible for your brain's memory function as well as for its emotional health.

Stress can wreak havoc on your moods - from the first second that you experience it. It can cause you to swing emotionally from feeling down or sad to feeling excited or happy.

It doesn't matter that the stress is not a reliable indicator of the circumstances that are actually going on in your life. It can create a false narrative because stress isn't felt in logic.

It's felt in the emotions. If you have a mood disorder, stress is different for you because stress can impact you to the point that you may find it difficult to function. But this stress on mood disorders doesn't just impact your life and make you struggle to get through the day.

It impacts what's known scientifically as your biological ageing. Everyone gets older in terms of going from birth to elderly. But that's the normal part of time passing and is known as chronological ageing as in one year follows the next.

Biological and chronological ageing are different. Stress affects mood disorders in a way that's different from normal ageing. This difference is what puts those who have mood issues at higher risk of getting diagnosed with a disease that's normally found in older people.

It's true that different health factors can cause faster biological ageing, but stress is the engine that drives the ageing when it's coupled with mood disorders and the risk factor is elevated.

Stress can speed up the ageing process when you have mood disorders because it alters the physical brain. It does this by changing the brain's white matter, which is in part how the brain uses and exchanges the information that it receives and gives.

Whether or not the changes are brought on due to the increased speed of stress related ageing are reversible depends on the length of time you're exposed to the stress and how severe it is.

Memory Lapses

Stressful experiences happen to everyone. You can go through things like relationship issues, the death of a spouse or a divorce. You may go through things like losing your job or experiencing a catastrophic illness or event.

Or you might not even experience big stressors at all. You might encounter small stresses, but over prolonged periods of time. One way to tell if you're stressed is to check your level of frustration.

That emotion goes hand in hand with stress. Regardless of the cause of the stress, studies have shown that stress changes the brain. Any time that the brain is changed, it can cause problems in several areas.

There can be problems with cognitive function, with communication and with moods. Stress speeds up the ageing process in the brain because it causes loss of cognitive function at a faster rate.

People who experience stress develop brain changes that have been linked with cognitive decline due to the acceleration of the biological age. These stress changes can mimic and then develop into early dementia as well as other brain function loss.

People who live with stress can begin to be forgetful earlier in life than the normal standard associated with ageing. Usually, those who struggle with memory issues chalk the lapses up to just being busy or being naturally or being forgetful.

They don't realize that their brain has undergone structural changes caused by stress. That's only one part of what goes on in the brain when stress runs rampant in your life. Another part is that stress impacts the brain's neurons.

There's a section within the brain that's dedicated to memory. Within this section of the brain, cells are developed. You need new brain cells in order to function well. Stress allows the continual release of these brain cells.

But it doesn't allow them to continue living - and you need healthy brain cells, because these are necessary for memory retention. Instead, stress actively kills brain cells, which impacts the emotional centre as well as the ability to recall and retain information.

As stress lingers, you'll begin to experience problems remembering what happened and your brain memory function can lose years off of its memory function. There are some questions as to how stress causes brain cells to die off and one theory is that it's due to the higher level of cortisol produced by someone who's under stress versus someone who isn't.

The bad thing about how stress speeds up the ageing process with memory lapses is that while some of it can be short term loss, it can also lead to long term memory lapses.

Weight Fluctuations

Stress causes changes in your weight. For some people, when they're under stress, they lose weight. This type of change can be caused from a difference in calorie intake from what they once ate.

Because of the stress, they lose their appetite and usually end up losing weight, sometimes rapidly. But it can also be caused because stress is forcing your metabolism to speed up.

On the flip side, stress can cause others to gain weight. This can be due to eating more calories in an attempt to deal with whatever it is that's stressing them. Either way that stress causes your weight to fluctuate, the bottom line is still that your body's metabolism is undergoing change.

Stress is extremely hard on your metabolism. One of the reasons that it causes people to put on extra pounds is because during stressful times, cortisol is released at higher levels than when you're not stressed.

Cortisol is responsible for increasing the desire to eat and specifically, it increases the desire to eat fattening or sugary foods. This metabolism changes and weight fluctuation impacts everything from your brain health to your muscles.

There is a link between stress, weight fluctuations, metabolism and the ageing process. Your metabolism naturally changes as you age. It's supposed to happen slowly with the passing of time.

But stress kick starts that metabolic change and forces your metabolism to change effective immediately. What that means for you is that stress is overwriting the natural stage that your body should be in with where it is metabolically.

It's making the structure, the molecular DNA of your body change - and not in a good way. It's adding year after year to your DNA - all within the space of months. During this process, it's giving you age related changes.

It's shaving off your life expectancy in leaps and bounds by skipping years and shortening your cells. As if that wasn't enough, it's introducing your body to health issues that are commonly associated with growing older, such as heart disease.

Weight fluctuations caused by stress break down your body's natural cell production and that revs up your biological age. While it's common to think that weight loss caused by stress from speeding up the metabolism is a good thing, it's not. When your metabolism speeds up, it creates oxidative damage, which in turn speeds up the ageing process.

Skin and Dental Problems

There's no doubt that stress isn't kind to your skin. When you're stressed, the body produces an abundance of cortisol. This hormone is known to destroy collagen. Collagen is the protein that keeps your tissues connected.

When it begins to age, you lose your youthful appearance. You'll experience wrinkles as well as sagging skin. It can also cause dry skin. When collagen is damaged, the skin begins to change, and it doesn't matter whether you're in your 20s or your 60s.

While it can be easy to think of skin in terms of what you see on the outside, it is actually what's going on inside the body that reflects on the outside of the body. When you're under stress, it causes issues like narrowing of the arteries due to high blood pressure.

In turn, a lack of the right amount of oxygen in your body impedes the saturation content for your skin. So you begin to develop problems like sagging skin, fine lines and more.
Stress ushers in premature wrinkles.

You can get them even if you're college age. It can even cause the colouring of your skin to change. You can develop these pigmentation changes because the stress is speeding up the normal ageing process that skin goes through.

Normally, your skin is supposed to regenerate. Old cells are sloughed off and new cells take their place. But when stress is at work, these processes are interrupted. New cells aren't produced in the quantity needed - just like what happens when you get older.

As the stress continues, the body is producing more cortisol, which leads to prominent veins, papering of the skin and more. You might even notice that your skin looks weathered and cracked.

What's taking place is that stress is speeding up your skin's ageing process. It's stripping you of years of soft, supple skin. Your skin isn't the only thing that's impacted by stress. It affects your teeth, too.

Stress causes pain in the face that can stem from the mouth. When you're under stress, you may grind your teeth. And it doesn't always happen when you're sleeping either. You may do it while you're awake and not even realize it.

It can cause you to lose tooth enamel as well as change the shape of your teeth. Both of those symptoms are what naturally happens when the body ages. When you grow older, teeth nerves change.

This change desensitizes the teeth, which in turn leads to oral problems because older people are often unaware that damage to the tooth is going on. This de-sensitivity in the nerves of the teeth can be triggered by stress, which can put you at higher risk for developing cavities.

No matter the level of care you take for your oral health, if you're under stress, it can cause gum disease. It can also cause mouth sores on the lips and inside the cheeks. These are a direct result of stress and are caused by biting at the inside of the lip or the inside of the cheek.

Substance Use and Abuse

Being under stress drives some people to use and abuse substances that harm their body. Family members of those who abuse substances are also under stress. There's a common understanding that when someone is under the influence, you're not dealing with the true person - but instead, you're dealing with whatever substance has been taken.

The same is true when it comes to the health and ageing process of someone who abuses substances. Their body isn't just dealing with the natural cause of ageing. They're synthetically ageing.

When someone abuses substances, it causes them to age inside and out at a faster rate, putting both their health and often, their lives at risk. As the body ages, normal cell changes take place that lead to issues associated with older people and the elderly.

With substance abuse issues, the stress starts that process, even if that person is young. From there, it leads to inflammation throughout the body. It also changes the way the brain is able to think, and it opens the door for the arrival of diseases.

Stress causes the acceleration of diseases that are brought on as a result of substance abuse. One of the reasons for this is because the substance often prevents the natural cycle of cell production.

It can cause heart disease from high blood pressure, stroke, and kidney disease. It affects every organ in the body - including the brain. The abuse can cause anxiety, depression and mental health episodes.

One reason behind this is because substance abuse can damage neurotransmitters in the brain. Many substances that are used can dry out the skin and rob you of important vitamin and minerals that you need - not just for skin health, but for organ health as well.

One of the things that happens as people get older is their vision begins to change, often worsening. Things like cataracts are common. When someone abuses a substance, it impacts the health of the eyes and can cause the biological age of the eyes to be decades older than what they are.

The veins are affected by stress. When stress speeds up the ageing process, it can cause the veins to widen. This can create long, thin red lines that stem out from the centre of a vein.

These veins can be large and can cover noticeable portions of the body wherever they develop, which is usually in the face or on the legs. This is a common side effect of substance abuse.

Losing patches of hair is also common with substance abuse. That's because the body's ageing process reaches the stage of someone who's much older. The reason that this happens is because the abuse interferes with the body's hair growth stage.

Instead of the hair following the growth cycle, then rest period naturally, the ageing process is sped up and the hair simply falls out faster than it grows. Therefore, people who abuse substances often look many years older than what they actually are.

Digestive Issues

Your digestive system is part of an elaborate system within the body and it works in tandem with the brain. When you're stressed by something, it can trigger a reaction in your gut.

Studies have shown that people who live with unresolved stress in their lives often experience temporary and sometimes life altering digestive issues. Your emotions can drive how your digestive system reacts.

Your brain decides what your digestive needs to do or not do and it uses neurons to communicate. When you're under stress, and you're feeling anxious or angry or sad, this information is relayed to the gut.

The stress that you feel then causes a reaction in this system and that reaction can be uncomfortable at best and make you physically ill at worst. Your body reacts to stress by limiting the amount of blood that travels to your digestive system.

It can make your stomach tighten up - even to the point of causing painful cramping. It can make you feel nauseated to the point you feel like you're going to vomit. Stress can cause a boost in the production of stomach acid, which makes you feel heartburn or sick to your stomach.

Long term stress often results in ulcers as a by-product of this over production of acid.

Stress can make you unable to have a bowel movement because you develop constipation, or it can lead to diarrhoea.

Stress can worsen certain digestive conditions such as IBS. It can also cause inflammation. You may experience an imbalance in the natural bacteria that's found in your gut.

Stress can affect your ability to eat the way that you usually do. Normally, when someone eats, the process of the food breaking down happens naturally and without incident.

But when stress is in the picture, it speeds up the ageing process in your digestive system and you develop issues that are common in older people. What ends up happening is you can develop a multitude of symptoms - including the same symptoms as someone who has diseases such as gastroparesis.

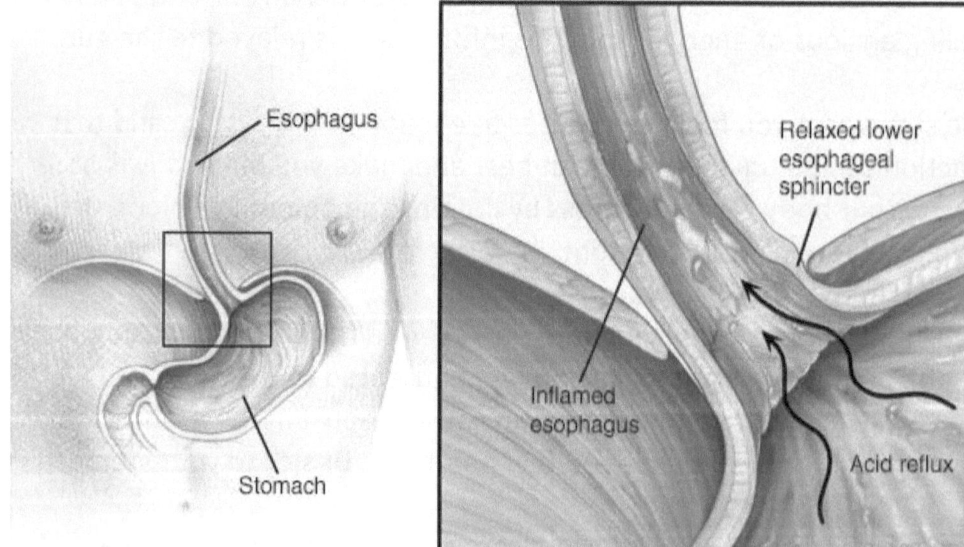

In this condition, the stomach doesn't empty like it's supposed to. Stress can cause slow emptying of the stomach. It can also lead to common digestive conditions associated with ageing such as flatulence, indigestion and even GERD. (**Gastroesophageal reflux disease**)

Stress isn't something you have to live with. In fact, it's a condition that can have serious side effects on you if you ignore it or learn how to merely live with it. Take control and reduce or eliminate stress that steals years off your life, starting now!

7 Rules for Reducing Stress and Improving Sleep

There's a strong correlation between how much sleep you get and how stressed you are. It's a vicious cycle that can cause mental distress and even wreak havoc on your physical well-being.

It's a well-known fact that people who don't get enough sleep are lethargic and constantly experiencing an energy slump. This causes irritability, which also makes it hard to fall asleep.

The reverse is also true. When you experience an exorbitant amount of stress during the day, it causes you to lie there awake – and that piles on more stress for the upcoming day.

The Huffington Post conducted a poll recently where they asked people what their number one stressor was. Lack of sleep was one thing that dominated the results. Stress and a lack of sleep combined can cause you to lose mental clarity and they can put more pressure on your body to perform at less than optimal standards.

So, it's vital that you learn how to implement stress relief measures that *also* work to lull you to sleep at night. When you wake up fully refreshed, you'll be able to tackle the world and anything it throws at you!

Rule #1 - Implement a Bedtime Technology Ban

If you want to toss and turn and have trouble getting (or staying) awake, just keep your cell phone right by your bed. For some of you, that won't be a problem – but for many people, it's become an addiction that disrupts their sleep routine and causes a lack of sleep.

Some people have their computer right beside the bed and the glow of it lights up the room at night. Ditto for notifications that come in on cell phones – sometimes with lights and sometimes with the inclusion of sounds.

Not only is it a physical factor, but it causes a certain amount of mental unrest when you're constantly checking emails or looking to see who posted what on Facebook.

The physical distraction of the computer glow tricks your body into thinking it's time for you to be awake. Your body won't produce the melatonin it needs and help you get (and stay) asleep, so you toss and turn all night.

Technology doesn't just have to be left out of the bedroom – it needs to be shut down quite a while before you go to bed. Your mind needs time to disconnect and wind down itself, and it can't do that if you're constantly feeding it information.

If you go to bed at 10 PM, try disconnecting around 8:30 PMM. Let your stress melt away and your mind relax. This isn't an easy habit to break, but you'll be able to implement it – even if you do it in baby steps, such as not taking it in the room with you, but using it right up until bedtime, and gradually creating a routine that's beneficial for your health.

Rule #2 – Adopt an Aromatherapy Habit

Aromatherapy soothes your mind and body for both sleep and de-stressing. Scents are a powerful element of our lives, and you can use the power of it to help you feel more rested.

Start off by choosing the right scents for you to unwind, let go of the anxiety the day brought, and get a good night's sleep. You don't want anything invigorating for bedtime – like peppermint.

That's a scent that's perfect to help you *start* your day – not end it. You want to look for scents that soothe and relax. Here are some possibilities:

- Bergamot

- Chamomile

- Jasmine

- Lavender

- Rose

- Vanilla

What's the best way to use these to unwind and get better sleep? You have many options when it comes to aromatherapy. You can find scented bath products (if you enjoy a bath before bed).

You can use candles, diffusers, wall plugins and more. Some people like to create or buy a special mist that they can spray on their pillows at night (or put on their wrists) before bed.

Rule #3 – Wind Down Your Day with Exercise

It sounds almost backwards – putting forth extra exertion when you really need to be relaxing and calming down. But that's just what exercise does for you! Exercise is a great stress reliever because it helps you release endorphins.

That's why you sometimes hear of athlete's bragging about their "runner's high" – because although they may start out fatigued, they hit a point in their regimen where the endorphins are released, and they feel good.

Feeling good is one of the first steps to you being able to sleep well tonight! Your body has probably been tensed and knotted up all day while you were at work. Allowing it to exercise gives you some relief – somewhere to pour all of that tension into.

Exercise also helps you sleep better at night. We joke as parents about letting our kids wear themselves out so they're ready for a good, long nap – but the same goes for us as adults!

When the Huffington post conducted a poll for people who exercise in terms of how they sleep, they discovered that people who exercise don't just get *more* sleep – they get *better* sleep.

As you might suspect, the harder you work out, the harder you snooze each night! If you're not used to exercising, start out slow and work your way up. You can start off with a simple 10-minute-a-day plan and increase it a bit each week.

The side effect of exercising to get better sleep and stress less is that you might shed pounds if you're overweight! Poor sleep makes people gain weight according to recent studies – and stress is a definite factor in consuming too many calories.

Try to exercise after work – plenty of time before bed, but in the evening. If you exercise too close to bedtime and you discover that you still feel restless, just move your exercise up to an early time.

Rule #4 – Let Bath Meditation Boost Your Sleep Count

For some people, bath time is their *only* time of the day when they unwind and kick stress to the curb. There are no clocks ticking, no technology vying for your attention, and nobody talking to you.

It's just you, your warm, soothing water, and whatever environment you've created to help you relax. The environment for your bath meditation is just as important as the sleeping environment you create.

If it's off, then you can't relax. A cold, sterile bathroom won't lend itself to a calming environment. You can use bath meditation whether you have a 10-minute bath or an hour-long bath.

Some people like to incorporate aromatherapy during their bath meditation – and you can find candles or bubble bath that soothes you with lavender or chamomile or any other scent that calms, rather than invigorates you.

Music is another option for you to consider. You can choose soft, relaxing music – or even invest in some sort of guided imagery CDs that will walk you through a visualization process that helps you meditate while in the bath.

Just as you've made the commitment to turn off technology at bedtime, do the same for your bath time, too. You can't really relax and meditate if your smart phone is ringing off the hook.

Make sure that when you ease yourself into your bath, you start to get familiar with how you're breathing. Most people go through each day using shallow breathing, and it's deep breathing that cleanses the stress from your body and helps you sleep better.

Let your mind wash away all of troubles and irritation of the day – picture it washing out to sea – and replace it with whatever the senses are experiencing at that very moment - the warmth of the water, the tranquil sounds, and the feeling of being unrestricted by ties or hosiery.

Everyone's different with how they meditate. Some like the guided imagery, while others want to have nothing to think about. Some like to use a mantra they can repeat throughout the meditation process. See what works best for you and then use that as your staple for better sleep and less stress.

Rule #5 – Become a Master at Time Management

During the Huffington Post surveys about sleep and stress, they noticed that most people started with phrases like, "Not enough time to…" Time is one thing we need more of and have less of in this day and age.

We have no time to relax. We push ourselves from the time our feet hit the floor in the morning right up until we go to bed – and we never get to bed on time. Instead, we give ourselves a minimal amount of sleep hours – and much of that is spent tossing and turning due to the stress of what all we couldn't accomplish in the day.

If you'll get firm with yourself and look at how much time you waste during the day, or how much time you're not as productive as you should be, then you'll free up more time for sleep.

Notice that didn't say, "free up more time to get tasks done." Many of you will learn new time management skills and forget to learn your lesson about sleep. Instead, you'll pack in more on your to-do list.

Keep a diary or journal of your daily routine. Notice all the times when you're surfing the web or standing around chatting with co-workers. That's time that you could be spending really accomplishing things so that once your day is done, you are rewarded with free time – "me time" – to pamper and nurture your body and mind.

You might also find that when you implement the other rules here, along with proper sleep hygiene, you'll be able to get more done throughout the day. That's because your mental clarity improves, and you tend to have more energy to tackle whatever the day may bring.

Rule #6 – Allow Deep Breathing to Replace Naps

There are some people who get in the habit of taking a daily nap – primarily because they've heard that power napping can help them achieve their goals for the day.

This might be true for many people. But if sleep eludes you, then naps could be causing the problem. A 10-minute power nap where you're basically just shutting your eyes and deep breathing is beneficial.

Going to bed for 2-4 hours in the middle of the day is a recipe for disaster. You'll never be able to go to bed at a regular bedtime and you'll lie there frustrated and annoyed that you can't go to sleep. It's a hard habit to break.

Try using deep breathing to energize yourself whenever you're in an afternoon slump. Breathe from your diaphragm and try to watch how often you're using shallow breaths throughout the day.

Rule #7 – Focus on Nutrition for Better Sleep and Less Stress

Foods are one area where what you eat can benefit or damage *both* your sleep and stress levels. If you want to alleviate stress and get better sleep, you need to limit or avoid alcohol and caffeine and eat foods that will help with both!

That means eating good protein like turkey or lean chicken, salmon, avocadoes, nuts Stress is what happens when you have so much to deal with emotionally or physically, and the burdens overwhelms you. Therefore, you can deal with many stressors and then all of a sudden something minor like dropping a glass of milk makes you start crying or feels like the final straw.

When you let stress build, it can feel as if it's all too much to handle so you end up doing nothing. Or worse, you start trying to deal with the stress by using alcohol or other unhealthy coping mechanisms. Dealing with stress head on is always best and here are a dozen ways that you can effectively do that.

Use Meditation

By using visualization or other forms of meditation, it can help relieve the pressure of stress building up. You don't have to be an expert to get started with meditation, either. You can use self-help books, online tutorials, guided imagery podcasts or other means.

Meditation takes your mind out of the middle of the stress and allows you to focus your thoughts. While you're meditating, the constant badgering you sometimes get from stress will be eliminated because it won't have centre stage in your thoughts.

This practice can be done anywhere at any time and it doesn't take long to reap the benefits of using meditation to deal with stress. Your mind and body will align and relax while using meditation.

It helps you let go of the negativity brought on by stress and instead keep your mind set on what's good, what's peaceful and what's helpful to you. Meditation gives you a coping skill that helps you eliminate the effects of the flight or fight response that occurs when you're under stress. You'll be able to lower your blood pressure and feel the weight of your stressors lift from your shoulders.

Know Your Stressors

Sometimes people aren't prepared for handling stress because they don't know exactly what it is about their life that's causing the stress reaction. By understanding what causes you stress, you can manage and eliminate it.

Fear and anxiety are a stressors. You can feel this kind of stress when you start playing the what if game - what if you lose your job, what if you can't your bills, what if your partner breaks up with you, what if you get sick, etc.

This is projection thinking that takes you out of the present day and causes your mind to live in a state of what "could" happen in the future. It's worrying about something that hasn't happened and may never happen.

Issues with relatives can also be a stressor. You could have people in your life that you simply don't get along with. Or you could have family members who are involved in situations that are bad and you feel the stress from that.

Leaving your normal way of life can be a stressor. This includes things like taking on a new job or leaving one, moving to a new home or new state, ending a relationship or starting one, going to college or graduating or having a child or having a child move out.

It's anything that shakes up how you routinely live your life. Health issues can be a stressor. Whenever you not feeling well or you're dealing with a chronic health problem, it can cause stress.

You feel the stress more when the health issue gets in the way of you being able to handle your day to day activities or your job. Job performance, both good and bad, can be a stressor.

When you do well at work, you may feel the stress and pressure to continually outdo yourself. When you do poorly, you may fear the boss's reaction or the loss of your job.
Work and family balance is another stressor.

You can feel pulled in two directions and feel like your life isn't balanced. This can cause you to feel stressed that you're not able to do your best at work or at home because your time is being stretched too thin.

Track Your Stressors

You can't fight what you can't see coming. But when you write down what you're going to be handling that day, it helps you deal with stress. It does this because you'll be identifying all the situations for that day and what the potential stressors are going to be.

Identify what it is about the situation (or the person) that's going to be in your day that's causing you to feel the stress. For example, if you have to attend your child's school for an event and the ex you don't get along with is going to be there, you should know ahead of time how to handle the negative emotions that will rise up.

Maybe you can strategize a way to minimize interaction, too. Know ahead of time that when you feel the anger, you'll practice meditation deep breathing exercises – because this can help you keep the situation and yourself calm.

Discover the Power of No

One common cause of stress is being too busy saying yes to others that you end up saying no to yourself. Know your limitations and don't exceed them. Every day you're going to be bombarded with people and situations that want you to say yes and give your time and energy.

But being a consistent "yes" person is the road to stress. You can't take time for yourself or what you really want to do if you don't practice using the power of no. Most people refrain from saying no out of fear that they'll appear selfish but saying no to someone isn't selfish.

It's practicing the art of self-care. When you have a problem telling other people no, or even telling yourself no to things, you add to your workload and can over-do what you're capable of.

You'll end up - not only stressed - but your immune system can take a hit as well since stress lowers your body's immune system defenses. Learning to say no can free you from the guilt that comes along with saying yes.

Many people only agree to something because they feel guilted into it or they guilt themselves into it. Just keep in mind that by saying no, you're taking care of your body and that's a good thing.

When you say no, let that be your one-word explanation. If someone asks, "why not" in response to your no, recognize that as a boundary issue. You don't owe anyone a reason. By saying no, you free yourself from overextending your own time and causing yourself unnecessary stress.

Get Enough Sleep

When you don't get enough sleep, it can cause a delayed reaction time in situations such as driving or trying to do your job. It also causes memory problems, weight gain, and can lead to serious health issues.

But not getting the right amount of sleep can cause stress and worsen the stress you may already have. A lack of sleep causes your decision-making ability to be affected and you end up making poor choices that increase your stress.

This happens when you get tired and you end up not really wanting to deal with whatever you're trying to handle. So, you end up saying no to good opportunities and yes to bad ones.

The lack of sleep can cause a cycle. When you don't get enough rest, it causes stress, which in turn causes insomnia. With each feeding into the other, it can make your stress level increase and reach the point where you find it difficult to deal with even minor problems.

Stop Ignoring Problems

You might believe that it's better not to deal with an issue that's causing you stress - that if you don't handle it, you're protecting yourself. But what you're doing is actually making your stress worse.

Common problems that people don't like to deal with, yet will cause stress are home repairs, car repairs, financial problems, children or teenage behaviour, arguments/issues with your spouse, family problems, environmental problems or fear of world problems.

When a problem arises, deal with it as soon as possible. If you put it off, the problem can only get bigger and when it grows, it'll take more of your energy and resources to fix.

Problems don't ride off into the sunset just because they aren't dealt with. They linger, quietly nagging at the back of your mind even while you're trying to ignore them. This internal nagging is at work building your stress. Face your problems, deal with them head on, and free yourself from stress.

Lower Your Expectations

One of the reasons that people have stress is because their expectations are out of whack. They have high expectations for other people and for themselves. So, when things don't work out as they expected, they feel not only disappointed, but stressed as well.

You can tell if your expectations are causing you stress if you think that your life wasn't supposed to turn out the way that it has - or if you think your partner wasn't supposed to behave the way he or she did.

It causes you stress because you were expecting something you didn't receive. You feel disappointment that the picture in your mind wasn't painted correctly in reality. Relief from stress is found by having realistic expectations for yourself and for the others in your life as well.

Learn to accept yourself for who you are, and others for who they are. When you consider your life, rather than feeling stressed for what hasn't worked out, focus on the good that has. Stop putting the pressure and stress on yourself to do more or to be more.

Find a Hobby You Enjoy

When you find something you like doing, it acts as a stress reliever because it gives you an outlet. A hobby can be a way for you to release the anxiety and pent up emotions that go along with dealing with stress.

You can get involved in music such as finding new songs or new bands. You can check out the local music scene where you live and attend free music festivals or shows for singers and bands just getting started.

Painting and other creative things such as sketching, or colouring can be a hobby that works as a stress outlet. There's also journaling. You don't have to be good at writing to journal.

It's just putting words down that are talking about how you're feeling or what's gone on during your day. Some people get into gardening. You can do vegetable and fruit or flowering gardening.

You can do a mixture of all three. Taking up knitting or crocheting is a great hobby that can help you deal with stress. You can learn a new skill such as a second language. Or you can learn how to play an instrument.

You can get involved in community theater or take acting classes. Going for regular hikes to explore new places is a great way to deal with stress. So is volunteering. By investing yourself in someone else, it successfully manages stress.

Create a To-Do List

You might wonder why creating a to-do list can help you manage stress. The answer is because when stress hits, you feel like everything is going wrong. You feel like nothing is within your ability to cope.

This feeling of being out of control can increase your stress level. Sometimes stress develops because people feel like they have so much to do or to overcome that it causes action paralysis, which then worsens stress.

By creating a to-do list, it helps a person prioritise the important things and they're able to focus on getting one thing at a time accomplished. Rather than focusing on what they have to do in its entirety, which can make stress rise, they're able to get through the day by choosing bite size action steps.

When you have a step-by- step to-do list it allows you to feel like you're in control. This works well even if you don't necessarily have a lot on your plate to handle. A physical list takes the pressure off your mental checklist.

like almonds or walnuts, and apricots (which soothe your muscles). Regular meals are key, too. You want your blood sugar levels stabilized so that you don't have to deal with mood swings and energy highs and lows.

12 Ways to Successfully Deal with Stress

Find Your Support System

One of the worst things about stress is when you try to keep it all inside. When your job isn't working out well, your partner isn't being helpful, and your kids are constantly pushing your buttons, you need a way to come to terms with the stress that you're feeling.

If you don't let it out, the stress pressure builds. You need to have someone to talk to about what you're going through. This someone may not be able to do anything to change your situation.

But by simply being there to listen, it relieves you of the buildup you're feeling. Talking through what's happening with you and what's causing your stress makes you feel better even if the situation is still present.

Your support can be a trusted friend, a relative, a romantic partner or a trained counsellor. Sharing how you're feeling relieves the emotional toll such as anxiety and depression that are often linked to stress.

Create a Strategy

Every single bit of stress in your life can be traced back to a trigger. It's always 'cause and effect'. Something happens and there's a mental, emotional or physical reaction. There are consequences or changes that led to the stress.

For example, your boss gives you a better position. You make more money. Now you're stressed. Not because you got the position that you wanted, but because there are more responsibilities.

It might be more time away from home. You might feel worried that you're not up to par.

What you have to do when stress hits, is trace backward to get to the root of your stress. When you find that, you can create a strategy to eliminate the stress.

If you take the new position at work, have a plan to enlist more help at home or hire outside help. If you're worried, you're not knowledgeable enough about the new position, ask for help such as more training or take a course. Your strategy should make you proactive and show you what you need to do to help you deal with your stress.

Let It Go

You must reach the place where you realize that despite how hard you try, there are some things you just can't solve. By wasting time worrying and trying to find a fix for the unfixable, you're just creating stress.

You can't fix a colleague who's lazy or is an idiot. You can't force a loved one not to break up with you. You can't order every event in your life to be as you wish it to be. You don't have any control over things that are outside your ability to change.

What you have to do is accept what you can't change and make peace with it. When you waste energy striving to try to force things to happen that are beyond your scope, you end up frustrated and stressed.

Accepting that you're powerless to change everything that affects you is a hard thing to do but it's necessary in order to deal with stress. It doesn't mean you're weak. It means you're strong enough to move on with your life rather than remaining stuck.

4 Ways to Slow Down the Ageing Process

As you get older, you start to notice some of the signs of ageing. One of the first changes that becomes apparent is that your skin starts to wrinkle, sag, and get drier. You may also notice that you put weight on in different places.

And as you age there are also changes in your joints that might make it more difficult for you to maintain your independence and mobility. You may also see changes in your mental health.

While you can't completely stop the ageing process, there are things you can do that will slow it down so that you can maintain your independence and live a full and happy life in your senior years.

Here we'll take a look at four areas where you can create a lifestyle that will slow the ageing process and support you in having a full life.

1 - Make Sure You're Getting the Right Nutrition

The earlier in life that you honor good nutrition the longer you can stave off the signs of ageing. Nutrition is critical to helping prevent disease and increasing your years of life. It can also help you to look and feel younger.

Antioxidants

It's important that you fill your diet with as many antioxidants as possible. These are chemicals that help your body to fight off environmental oxidation that can lead to faster ageing.

Antioxidants are found in high amounts in these foods:

- Blueberries
- Broccoli
- Green including kale, spinach, turnip, and mustard greens
- Strawberries
- Tomatoes
- Apples
- Red grapes
- Beans

While these are foods that have a high concentration of antioxidants, they can be found in a wide variety of foods. You'll especially find antioxidants in fruits and vegetables, but some are even found in meat, poultry, and whole grains.

Avoid Processed Foods

If you eat a diet that consists of foods that aren't processed including fruits, veggies, lean meats, dairy products, and whole grains you'll be in the best shape.

Processed foods, on the other hand, contain little or no nutrition and often are high in calories from sugar, salt, and fat. You'll want to avoid eating processed foods as much as possible. Processed foods contain:

- White flour
- White sugar
- Trans fats
- Artificial colours
- Artificial flavours
- Preservatives
- Artificial sweeteners

These are all things you'll want to avoid in order to slow down the ageing process. These foods cause your body to experience inflammation, which is responsible for weight gain, joint problems, ageing skin, and the increased risk of disease.

If you follow the simple advice to eat "real" food that hasn't been processed, you'll have fewer signs of ageing and better health.

2 - Implement a Proper Skincare Regime

Skincare is essential to slowing down the ageing process. This is the first thing you notice and the first sign to others of your age. It's important to note that good nutrition is the first step toward healthy, younger skin.

Exercise

Regular exercise is actually good for your skin and can slow down ageing. That's because when your body gets heated up, blood rushes to the surface of your skin to let heat escape.

Having more blood flow to your skin actually helps it to become rejuvenated and get the nutrients it needs. Even just walking for 30 minutes a day will help you get this effect.

Hydration

Your skin needs moisture in order to prevent wrinkles and other signs of ageing. It's critical that you drink a lot of water to keep your body hydrated. Your body always distributes nutrients to vital organs first and then to the more peripheral areas of the body.

If you don't drink enough water, your skin will be one of the first places that gets deprived of water. This causes the cells to shrink and can lead to wrinkles and dry skin.

Three Skincare Steps

Hydration comes from within the body, but you also need to add moisture externally to your skin. As you age, you'll want to maintain a skincare routine that includes gentle cleansing, exfoliation, and moisturising.

You may need to cleanse your face only once a day if it gets drier. The best time to cleanse is at the end of the day to remove makeup, dirt, and oils that have accumulated throughout the day.

You also need to make sure that you exfoliate. This is a process of removing dead skin cells from the surface of your skin. When you exfoliate, you actually allow your moisturizer to penetrate more deeply into healthy tissue.

You can use a scrub with particles to help remove dead skin cells. This process is called mechanical exfoliation. You can also use chemical exfoliation with products that contain retinols.

These acids help to dissolve dead skin cells and are found in many anti-ageing formulas. You'll also want to look for a moisturizer developed for ageing skin. Many moisturizers contain antioxidants and retinols to further slow ageing.

Get Plenty of Protection from the Sun

Damage from the sun is one of the most powerful causes of ageing skin and skin cancer. The younger you are when you protect yourself from the sun, the better. But even if you're already ageing, it's not too late to protect yourself from the sun.

Look for products that contain at least SPF 15. These will give your skin protection from harmful UV rays in the atmosphere. When you're outside for long periods of time, look for areas of shade that will protect you.

Wearing a hat and appropriate clothing will also protect your skin from sun damage.

3 - Give Yourself a Mental Health Makeover

Many people battle depression as they age. But this shouldn't be considered a normal condition for people who are ageing. Some factors that lead to depression in seniors include:

- Chronic disease
- Social isolation
- Death of a spouse or family members

If you're struggling with feelings of hopelessness and sadness, it's important that you seek help from a professional as soon as possible. There are many things you can do to improve the way you feel.

Staying social is one critical element of good mental health. Joining groups that allow you to spend time with others is a great way to boost your spirits and provide you with positive mental health.

If you suffer from a chronic disease, a support group may be able to help you feel better about your condition. It's also important to practice self-care and ask for help and support when you need it.

Often people have the misconception that it's normal to feel depressed or blue when they get older. Because of that they either don't seek help or get misdiagnosed. Make sure that you don't just dismiss your feelings as a normal part of ageing.

Beyond depression, seniors also experience mental health issues such as:

·   Dementia
·   Anxiety
·   Problems with sleep

The best way to slow down problems with mental health is to take good care of your body at the youngest age possible. Nutrition and exercise are critical for maintaining good mental health.

It's also important to accept new challenges that require strategic thinking. Even completing puzzles can help you to stay mentally sharp.

You also want to make sure that you avoid social isolation and make it a point to participate in social activities. You may also find it beneficial to seek spiritual connection through a faith community.

4 - Making Sure You Maintain Your Mobility

One of the biggest concerns for someone who's getting older is mobility. You may be worried that you won't be able to get around the way you once did. Some causes of mobility problems include:

·   Muscle weakness
·   Arthritis
·   Vision problems
·   Medication use

- Heart disease
- Balance problems related to stroke

Many problems with mobility can be prevented by taking good care of your body with nutrition and exercise. The more activity you get, the more mobile you'll likely be in your senior years.

It's also important to treat vision problems that might make it difficult to move properly. Sometimes just by changing your glasses prescription or getting treatment for cataracts you can return to normal mobility.

If you experience muscle weakness or balance problems, you should always check with your doctor. An adjustment in medication could be all that you need. But if medication isn't the problem, exercise could be the solution.

Weak muscles can be strengthened. Even in your senior years you can begin a fitness routine that includes aerobic activity and strength training. Working your muscles will help to prevent fractures and allow you to move freely.

Make sure to talk with your doctor before beginning a fitness routine to make sure it's appropriate for you. But in most cases, it will be appropriate to take a walk each day and to lift some light weights for your upper body.

Just these simple steps can slow the ageing process and help you to remain independent for a long time. Ageing doesn't have to mean giving up the things you love to do.

5 Best Anti-Ageing Exercises

As we age, hormonal levels diminish and our skin, muscles and bones begin to deteriorate. A good anti-ageing exercise regime should stimulate hormone production and promote strength and flexibility.

Studies have shown that nothing works better to attain anti-ageing effects than a regular exercise program. 'Regular' is the key word – unless your exercise program is consistent, the process won't have the same effect.

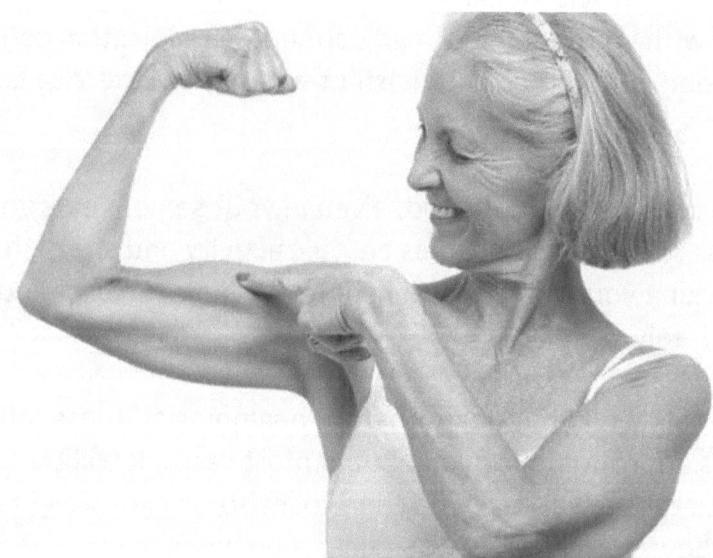

There are certain types of exercises that will help you stay active, live a longer and happier life and stay mentally alert. How often and how strenuous you make your exercise program depends on your personal needs, both physical and your daily lifestyle.

The Best Exercises to Reap Anti-Ageing Results

There are three definitive types of exercises that are best suited for an anti-ageing regime:

- **Flexibility** – The most important exercises to beat the ageing process. It increases blood circulation and releases serotonin, which is a chemical produced by the brain and is necessary for overall health and well-being. Flexibility exercises are also safe and easy to perform.

- **Strength Building** – These exercises will help build sturdiness and sustain bone mass. Your chances of having a debilitating injury are lessened as you build your muscle strength. Exercises to improve the muscles in your shoulders, back and legs will also help with hormone production.

- **Cardiovascular** – Designed to keep your heart healthy, aerobic exercises also help fight depression and keep your weight down. Running, brisk walking and any other exercise that will increase your heart rate for a sustained period of time release brain chemicals that produce hormones.

Research has shown that there's no particular time of the day when exercising is best, however accidents seem to happen more often in morning hours – muscles and joints seem to be less flexible at that time.

Preferably, exercise when you aren't too tired, but when you've been up and about for a while.

Mid-afternoon seems to be a good time for most people to perform exercises without too much fear of injury.

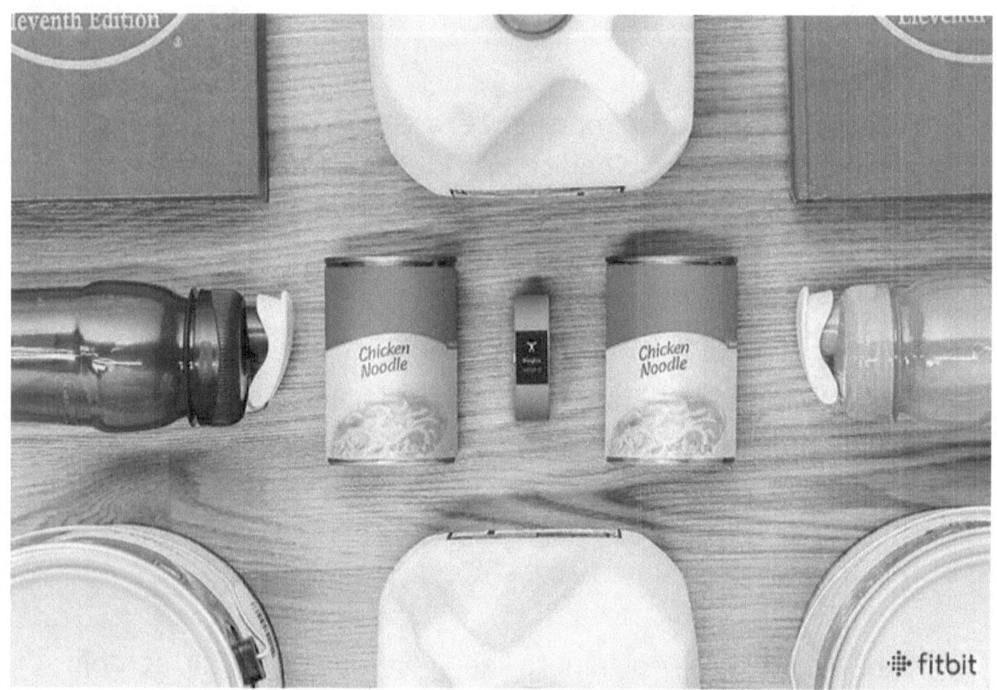

Picture courtesy of Fitbit

You don't need a home gym or an expensive membership in a gym.

One piece of equipment that you know you'll use on a regular basis is the best investment is one that you know you'll use on a regular basis.

Your kitchen or garden shed has many items that would be suitable for lifting as weights, stepping up and down etc.

You could fill a plastic milk container with sand, soil or even cement as well as water. This will make great small weights.

7 Things You Can Do to Look Younger

Men and women are frantically searching for "Fountain of Youth" remedies to make them look as young as they can.

Unfortunately, many are choosing medical treatments rather than searching for more healthy alternatives.

There are some things you can do to look younger besides opting for injections of Botox or invasive surgeries like liposuction and facelifts.

Look below at some of the "gentler" ways to seem younger than you really are:

1. **Dress Your Age** – Almost nothing makes you look older than you are than attempting to dress in the same style of clothing that your daughter or granddaughter wears. Dress your age and appear younger than you are.

2. **Sleep Your Way to Youth** – Your best sleep happens during what is called the "rejuvenation hours." Your face won't reveal as many lines and your eyes won't be as puffy. If you're in a habit of waking up at 3 or 4 o'clock in the morning, try meditation or take the natural herb, melatonin before turning in for the night.

3. **Your Diet Can Make You Younger** -- Obesity can become a problem as you grow older because of a slower metabolism. Keep your weight on track, make your skin glow and your blood healthy by eating foods with beneficial properties.

4. **Exercise Regularly** – Nothing benefits your overall health like having an exercise regime that you enjoy and perform on a

regular basis. No matter what exercise you choose, getting your body moving can drop the years from your body and mind.

5. **Use Makeup Sparingly** – You'll appear to be much younger than you really are if you use makeup more to enhance your natural assets rather than attempting to cover up the flaws. Get a professional makeup artist to show you how to apply your makeup in the best and most flattering way.

6. **Choose the Proper Hairstyle** – Are you still wearing the same style you had in the 70s – or is your hair dull or grey? Do yourself a favour and visit a professional hairstylist and let him or her design a style that fits your face and colouring.

7. **Break Those Bad Habits** – If you smoke or drink too much alcohol, cut down or quit if possible. Too much alcohol will dry out your skin and smoking will rapidly age your entire body.

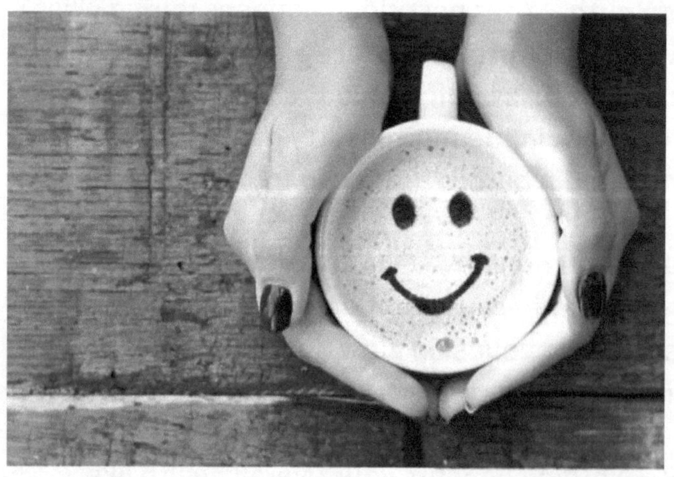

In your quest to look and feel younger, don't forget your "attitude."

Do what you can to keep yourself upbeat and positive – and for goodness sake,

don't forget to smile!

Defy the Ageing Process with a Positive Mental Attitude

Perhaps the most important thing you can do for yourself to increase longevity and live a happier, healthier life is to learn how to develop and keep a positive mental attitude.

The process of developing an attitude that will help you later in life should be nurtured during the younger years. How you learn skills when you're young to help cope with adversities and strategies through life will become all important when you reach a time that requires those skills.

We now know how important it is to our mental health to figure out a mission for our lives. Then, as you go through the stages and hurdles of life, you can reassess that mission and reconfigure it for where you currently are on life's path.

Living a full, rich life should be a goal that you not only strive for but work toward by doing everything possible to make sure you're healthy, both in body and mind to withstand the ravages of time.

The Most Important Tools to Keep a Positive Attitude

Scientific research indicates that "retirement" as our ancestors viewed it really isn't a good thing for us to keep a positive mental attitude about life. Below are some helpful tools for you to live by if living a full, rich life is of concern to you.

- **Keep Busy** – A rocking chair isn't the way to achieve "Fountain of Youth" effects during the ageing process. We now know that keeping active, both in body and mind is the best way to live a long and productive life.

- **Write Your Own Road Map** – Baby boomers entering their 60s never expected to age, so they're now looking for ways to keep their youth – but most are trying to retain their youth with cosmetic surgery, pills or surrounding themselves with youthful "things" such as a bright red sports car.

Writing your own road map for the rest of your life is empowering and can also   help to build your mental aptitude just as you would build your muscles through exercise.

- **Cultivate Healthy Relationships** – The relationships you cultivate with family and friends can make the difference in how you view the rest of your life. Taking trips and learning new things are all better done with someone you care about than alone.

Take the necessary steps to develop a positive mental attitude that will help you through the ageing process gently and optimistically.

Is There a Therapeutic Remedy for Ageing?

As far as anyone knows, there is no magic pill to keep your youth intact forever, and if there is, nobody is telling!

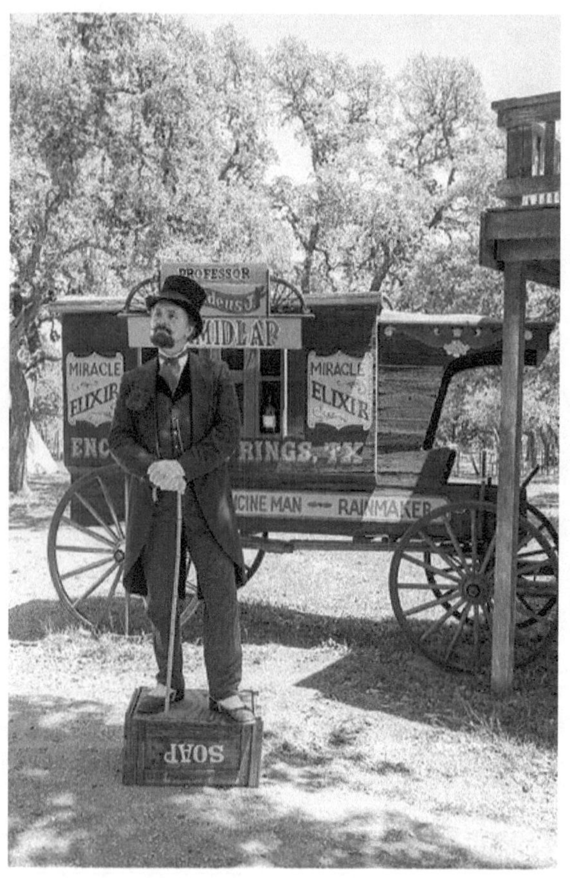

There is however a lot of hype about how taking a pill or sipping a concoction will restore your energy, build your muscles and help you lose weight.

Don't believe the hype.

All you will ever get for your money and time is the possibility of developing a real health problem and probably look much older through illness.

But while there isn't a single remedy to reverse the effects of ageing, there are ways to help keep the ageing process at bay and improve your health and lifestyle. If you're hoping to turn back the clock, talk to your doctor and do some research yourself before taking a pill or drug that's said to be a sure-fire way to regain your youth.

The Evidence is Now in on Anti-Ageing Therapies

While there's no tried and tested method of warding off the ageing process, there are proven therapies that can preserve your general health and extend your life expectancy.

Below are some therapies that you may want to check out:

- **Hormone Therapy** – Hormones are natural chemicals produced in your body. As you age, hormonal levels decline, and the ageing process becomes more pronounced.

  Restoring those levels with therapies such as DHEA (Dehydroepiandrosterone) and HGH (Human Growth Hormone) may slow ageing, boost immunity and improve cognition capability.

Hormone therapy can come with its own set of problems, such as liver damage. Check with your doctor before you begin any type of hormone therapy.

- **Antioxidants** – "Free radicals" (the substance your body produces as it processes the food you eat) can be one cause of ageing and diseases.

  Antioxidants such as the vitamins and minerals contained in the food you eat can neutralize these free radicals and prevent diseases like diabetes and heart disease.

If you are not eating a balanced diet, you might benefit from vitamin supplements such as Vitamin B6, C, E and A.

- **Restrict Your Caloric Intake** – Recent studies have found that reducing the number of calories in your diet can help you live a longer, healthier life.

  You must be sure that you are getting enough nutrients such as those found in fruits and vegetables.

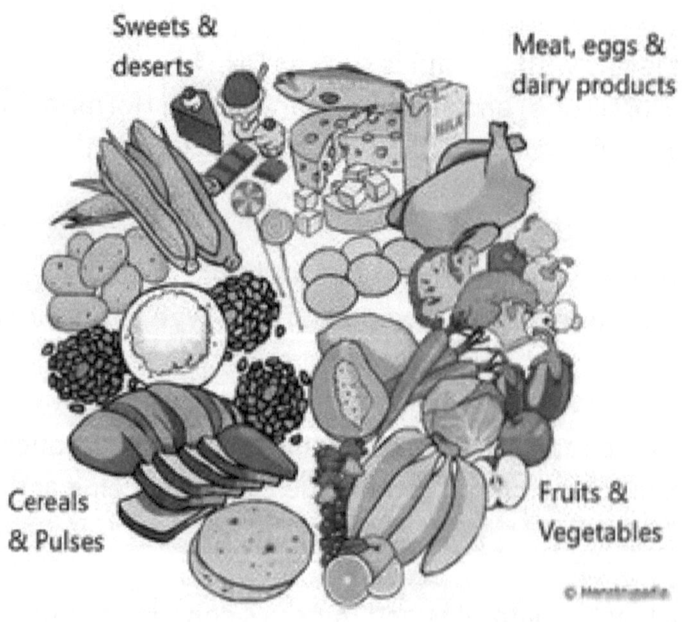

There are many factors involved in the ageing process, and what may be effective for one, might not be healthy for another.

Be sure and talk to your doctor before you begin any type of therapeutic remedy.

Over 40 Skin to Die For

Is it all in the genes – or can we do anything to prevent the deep lines and dry skin from ageing us prematurely? In our youth we felt our baby-soft skin was invincible, and we spent hours basking in the sun and tanning our bodies to a golden-brown hue.

Now, some of us – over 40 – are paying dearly with skin that's turning to leather before our very eyes. What can be done, if anything, to get back some of that youthful glow and elasticity?

We need to know that there are two types of ageing that affects our skin – intrinsic (genes) and extrinsic (external reasons, such as exposure to the sun's rays). While some deterioration of the skin goes along with the ageing process, there are ways we can lessen its effects. These include:

- **Minimizing repetitive facial expressions** – Frowning, smiling or raising your brows repeatedly can cause those deep furrows around your eyes and mouth and across your forehead.

- **Sleeping positions** – Do you sleep with your face pressed into the pillow or with the side of your face resting on the pillow? If you do, chances are you'll eventually discover "sleep lines" across your chin and cheeks. Try to sleep on your back to minimize this type of wrinkle.

- **If you smoke – quit** – Smoking can cause unsightly lines and wrinkles, not to mention a yellowish, leathery texture to your skin. When you quit smoking the lines and unhealthy coloring and texture will immediately begin to disappear.

- **Wear sunscreen** – Sunscreen should be worn daily and become part of your overall skin protection regime. Be sure you choose a broad spectrum (UVA and UVB) protector and at least 15 or higher SPF.

While you can't really do anything about the intrinsic (genetic) factors that contribute to ageing skin, you can opt for a medical treatment such as dermabrasion, chemical peeling, botulinum or injectable fillers.

Newer treatments such as radiofrequency are taking the place of more invasive procedures like a complete facelift.

See a qualified dermatologist (To become a Dermatologist in the UK, you will need to have completed a degree in medicine recognised by the General Medical Council, as well as a two-year foundation programme which specialises in **Dermatology**). if you suffer anxiety over ageing skin or just want to look and feel younger. There are newer and better treatment options becoming available all the time, and your dermatologist should be able to suggest a treatment for you and your type of skin.

Anti-Ageing Moisturisers – Creams v. Serums

With the demand for anti-ageing skin care products at an all-time high, manufacturers are constantly evolving their methods of delivering dewy, youthful skin.

Anti-ageing creams are the standard - a hybrid formula based on the tried and true moisturizers.

Most of us would think Nivea was one of the oldest brands, or Ponds Cold Cream. However, the world's oldest cosmetic face cream was revealed recently when archaeologists opened a 2,000-year-old capsule found at a Roman site in the heart of London.

The newer product is the serum, an over-the-counter variation on products that were initially used by aestheticians and dermatologists for advanced skin care. Now you can buy either type at prices ranging from department store to discount store levels.

Creams are soothing, rich and designed to provide the extra moisture that ageing, sun exposure and environmental toxins steal from the skin over time. No longer the big generic jar on your grandmother's dresser that went on the whole body from face to toes, today's anti-ageing creams are specially designed for the face and neck.

Creams also come in formulas that are suitable for dry, oily or combination skin types. Choosing a cream for your skin is extremely important. Retinal - the Vitamin A derivative - is found in creams at all price points.

Naturally the more expensive creams have a larger amount of retinal A than the lower-priced products. Aloe Vera, Vitamin E and grape seed oil are also popular additives in anti-ageing cream moisturizers. Cream moisturizers for daywear need to have a high sun protection factor (SPF), while night creams don't need this feature.

Serums are getting much attention in the anti-ageing market for their claims of faster, visible results than creams can deliver. As with anti-ageing creams, the key ingredients in most serums are Retinal (Vitamin A) and peptides.

It's the delivery of peptides that are rapidly absorbed into the skin that gives the notable changes. Peptides act on the collagen levels, which make the skin appear fuller and cause wrinkles to be less apparent.

Continuous use of these serums is absolutely necessary to stimulate collagen production. Erratic use of serums won't sustain visible results. Top quality serums tend to cost more than creams.

Some serums have a two-step process compared with cream that you simply apply to the face. Another claimed advantage for serums is the inclusion of an ingredient – argireline - which works on the skin much like Botox, it is sometimes called Botox in a jar. But, without the toxins. In fact, they work very differently.

Argireline is claimed to be a safe way to relax the muscles, which smoothes out wrinkles. Serums with high concentrations of this element claim up to 25% reduction in fine line and wrinkles after 30 days of continuous use. Argireline is also said to reverse sun damage effects on skin.

Argireline prevents the formation of expression wrinkles (laughter lines and crow's feet) by inhibiting muscle movement.

Our muscle contracts because a super lipid (called a vesicle) and releases a neurotransmitter to the synapses, (a junction between two nerve cells, consisting of a minute gap across which impulses pass by diffusion of a neurotransmitter.) sending a signal for the muscle to move. For simplicity our brain zaps across the gap, causing a cascade of expansion/contraction or ripples.

Three proteins, called the SNARE complex, have major roles in the final stages of this process (called exocytosis).

Argireline is made by a company based in Barcelona, Spain, called Lipotec.

They discovered that acetyl hexapeptide mimics one of the proteins in the SNARE complex and as a result can make it unstable.

Even if a SNARE is slightly unstable it won't work.
No SNARE means there is no muscle movement.
No frowning means there are no wrinkles (despite the fact that there are many other ways that wrinkles are caused).

The only independent study that I have found was conducted by a Spanish university and published in the **International Journal of Cosmetic Science** that says that a 10% concentration of Argireline reduced wrinkles by 30% over 30 days.

The choice of creams versus serums for anti-ageing skincare is largely an issue of cost and ease of use.

One way to get the best of both worlds at a price savings is to use a serum for several months to achieve the desired wrinkle reduction and then switch to an anti-ageing cream.

If that works well to sustain your visible skin improvements, then you have a combination skincare regime at a lower average cost. You can add back the serums for a month several times a year to boost results.

Or, you can conduct your own comparison. Use a serum for 30 days and take a close-up photo of the results. Then switch to a cream for the next 30 days and take a photo of the skin.
Compare these closely to see whether serum or cream is the best anti-ageing skincare product for your skin, your budget and your daily cosmetic routine.

War on Wrinkles

If you have wrinkles, you might want to get rid of them at any price. Some may like their 'laughter lines'.

If you don't have wrinkles, you may *make* some appear just by worrying about how to avoid them!

This whole exaggerated fear of wrinkles is a cosmetic surgeon's dream come true. They'll inject you with something that could kill in high enough doses - just to smooth out a few lines on your face, and then it's only temporary!

You will have to go back month after month and pay a small fortune just to keep those signs of ageing away. Before you know it, you're paying more for maintenance on your wrinkles than it costs to keep your car serviced.

You can take control of your wrinkle management regime with simple, low cost, natural approaches.

Here are some tips to help keep ageing at bay:

- Drink 6-8 glasses of water a day. It almost sounds too simple, but it's very important to hydrate from the inside-out. Your skin is the largest organ of your body and it desperately needs to be hydrated. Drinking water, not lattes or sodas, keeps your skin supple and the rest of your body benefits, too!

- Increase your intake of fruits and vegetables. The natural antioxidants in these fresh foods help strength skin tissue so that it repairs and rebuilds on schedule.

> Fresh vegetables are often transported great distances after being harvested, this makes them less nutritious than frozen vegetables. So, if you don't have access to quality raw vegetables, then frozen may be a better choice nutritionally speaking

- Take vitamin and mineral supplements - particularly skin-friendly Vitamins A, C, and E. It doesn't matter how many creams you put on your skin - if your body isn't well-nourished, hydrated and supported with vitamins, signs of ageing will show up and cause damage to your appearance.

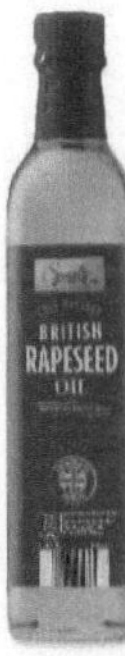

- Include more nuts and oils in your diet. Use high quality virgin or extra virgin olive oil in your salads and for cooking.

Snack on walnuts, peanuts or almonds.

These foods help your body lubricate the skin from the inside-out.

Take a serious look at rapeseed oil and nutritional benefits.

Most of us are aware of olive oil's health benefits the associated Mediterranean diet. However, fat too many people are unaware of the nutritional benefits of rapeseed oil, such as that it contains less saturated fat than all other cooking oils and fats – fifty percent less than olive oil.

It is therefore high in unsaturated fats, particularly mono-unsaturated, and replacing saturated fats with these has been shown to reduce cholesterol, which is good for heart health. It is also a rich source of vitamin E.

- Additional antioxidants can be applied to the skin with creams made from soy protein, Vitamin A (retinol), peptides, hyrodxy acid and CoQ10 Enzyme.

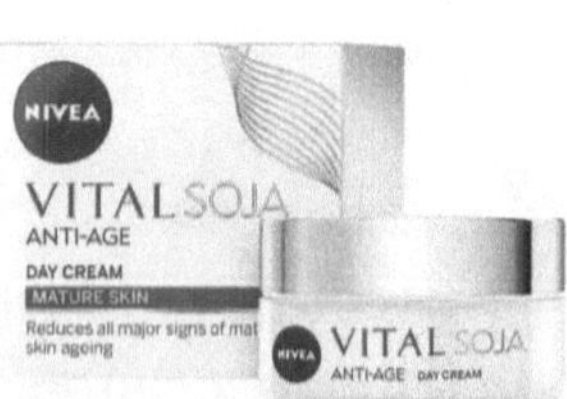

These are not cheap, but you may get better quality with brands from health shops than some of what you could buy for twice the price in a department store or supermarket. And the natural products aren't filled with artificial chemicals.

Combating wrinkles is an inside job as well as outside maintenance regime. No amount of expensive designer creams will overcome what your body lacks to rebuild damaged cells.

Inexpensive Anti-Ageing Eye Creams You Can Make

It's not just women, but men too have a desire to look young and the cosmetic industry is making a fortune from the demand.

Consumers are looking for the chemical or natural equivalent to the fountain of youth. Young and older use anti-ageing skin care products.

In fact, the earlier you start taking care of your skin, the less damage you will have to undo later. Because of the high consumer demand, anti-ageing products are sometimes expensive.

It's important to be a savvy shopper when it comes to looking for less expensive anti-ageing products, because cheaper brands on the shelves at discount shops often only contain a fraction of an anti-ageing element that's more concentrated in the high-priced products.

What if you want to take care of your skin, but your budget just doesn't stretch for monthly refills of the expensive, department store brands? You can make your own natural, organic anti-ageing skincare formulas at home.

The best ingredients come from nature, not a chemistry lab. You probably have many useful items right in your kitchen! Here are a few ideas:

- **Apple and Potato Soothing Eye Cream** – Grate a medium sized potato using a fine grater. Add in 3-4 tablespoons of unsweetened applesauce from the supermarket (or make your own if you're extra industrious) and mix well. Allow the mixture to chill for 5 minutes in the fridge. Then take a small spoon and gently apply the mixture around your eyes. Recline and place a damp cloth over the eyes. After 5 minutes, rinse off the mixture with water. Repeat this process at least once a week.

- **Vegetable Medley Eye Circle Cream** – Not only are vegetables good for your body from the inside, but they're also good for your skin from the outside!

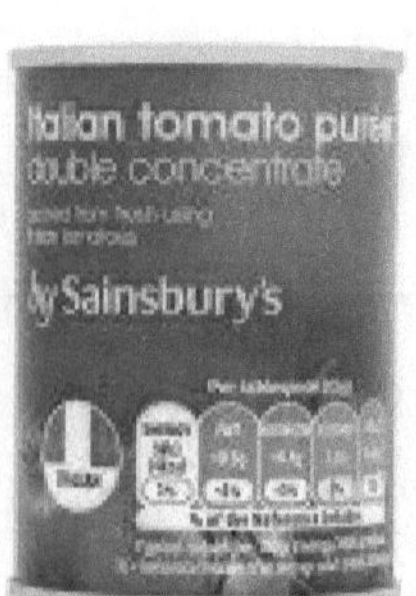

Combine a half-cup of tomato puree (canned from supermarket it good, Sainsbury's 35p), a pinch of turmeric powder, and one tablespoon of lemon or lime juice. Stir in wheat flower until a paste is formed. Form the paste around your eyes and let it dry there for 10 minutes as you recline. Gently rinse away the paste, being careful not to pull on the delicate skin around your eyes. Repeat weekly or anytime you feel fatigued and need to look refreshed.

- **Herbal Tea Bags** – All you have to do is place an herbal tea bag in warm water until it's soaked, and then place the tea bags over your eyes with a soft cloth over the tea bags while you lie down for 10 minutes. Tea has healing properties for your skin. Chamomile is a favourite for skin refreshment, but you can also choose other types.

Each of these homemade anti-ageing skincare eye treatments is simple to prepare, inexpensive and uses products that are easily found at the supermarket or in health food shops.

Total Body Rejuvenation

What do celebrities do when they are stressed out? they head for expensive spas to get pampered, nourished and refreshed.

If your budget is more inclined towards a run in the park and a smoothie to refresh yourself, then you have to take charge of your own wellness. And really, that's the best approach anyway!

Don't wait until your body is screaming for help with aches, pains, wrinkles or stress. Real anti-ageing is proactive and starts well before the first signs of ageing appear. Most of what you need to look and feel great at any age is in the health food shop - or your own kitchen!

Green Tea is calming and delicious, but it also has so many curative properties that it's practically a health care centre in a tiny tea bag. Green tea has been shown in some studies to reduce the risk of breast cancer, colon cancer and gastrointestinal cancer.

It's also calming if you have Crohn's disease or Irritable Bowel Syndrome. Green tea is also shown to be effective in protecting against heart disease and improving mental alertness. Drink one or two cups of green tea daily for maximum benefits.

Ginger is an old-fashioned remedy for travel sickness that's usually taken in a capsule form. Recent studies show that ginger or ginger extract can help calm irritable bowel syndrome, morning sickness, nausea and migraine headaches.

Cranberry juice is another home remedy for urinary tract infections. Drinking cranberry juice regularly helps keep away painful infections and protects against Type II Diabetes.

Turmeric is a seasoning found among the spices. Not only is this flavourful for cooking but it's also shown to have a positive effect on Rheumatoid Arthritis, bursitis (joints), osteoarthritis and lower back pain.

Olive Oil is useful in cooking and salad dressings, but the little olive is more powerful than you know. Olive oil or olive extract combats fungus and yeast infections, bacterial infections and the pesky bugs that bring on colds.

These are easy to incorporate into your menu plans for maximum effect. It can be as simple as adding more Turmeric in your cooking or choosing to relax with a cup of Green Tea instead of a fizzy drink.

Anti-Ageing Energy Boosters

Remember when you were a child and you had to get booster jab to protect against certain diseases? That booster was necessary because the effect of the first jab simply did not last a lifetime.

The same with anti-ageing. You can't just do something once, and then expect it to last forever.

There is no point in banging the drum that time, environment and gravity take a toll on our skin and body. Periodically, you will need some anti-ageing energy boosters.

Keep wrinkles at bay and your energy level tank filled to the rim with these tips:

1. **Get out of your house**! You need fresh air and hopefully some sunshine regularly. This doesn't mean getting a suntan, but if the sun is out, use a high number SPF sunscreen to avoid skin damage from ultraviolet rays. And don't stay outdoors during the mid-afternoon hours when the sun is most powerful. Go out in the morning and late afternoon.

NHS says:

Do not rely on sunscreen alone to protect yourself from the sun. Wear suitable clothing and spend time in the shade when the sun is at its hottest.

When buying sunscreen, the label should have:

- a sun protection factor (SPF) of at least 30 to protect against UVB
- at least 4-star UVA protection

UVA protection can also be indicated by the letters "UVA" in a circle, which indicates that it meets the EU standard.

Make sure the sunscreen is not past its expiry date. Most sunscreens have a shelf life of 2 to 3 years.

Do not spend any longer in the sun than you would without sunscreen.

2. **Reduce the heat inside your home**. Keeping the temperature too warm causes the air to dry out, which is as bad for your breathing as it is for your skin. Plus, you're more likely to be lethargic in a room that's too warm. If you're slightly chilled, reach for a sweater instead of the thermostat.

3. **Cut down sugar**. Sugar is no more a cure for fatigue than petrol is useful in extinguishing a fire. When you need a quick snack, choose protein, fruit, nuts or seeds. You'll get more energy without the sugar rush and sugar crash that's so draining.

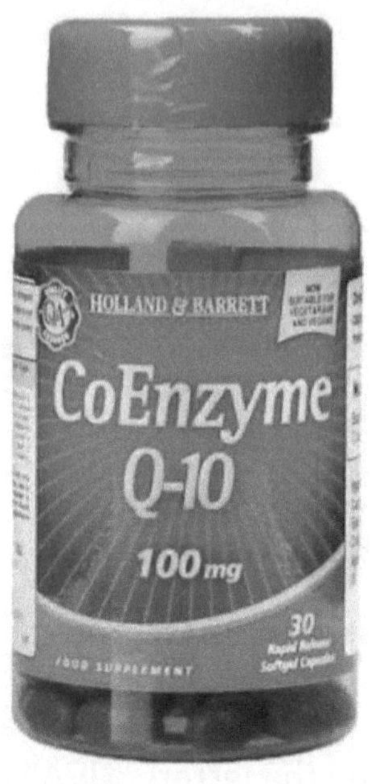

4. **Divide your daily supplements**.

Take part of your vitamins and minerals in the morning and the remainder in the evening. That way, your body has a more consistent level of support all day.

Coenzyme Q10 is a great natural energy booster without the damageing properties of hyper-caffeinated, so-called *energy* drinks.

Coenzyme Q10, also known as CoQ10, is a compound that helps generate energy in our cells.

Our body produces it naturally, but its production tends to decrease with age. However, you can get it through supplements or foods.

Health conditions like heart disease, brain disorders, diabetes, and cancer have been linked to low levels of CoQ10

Plenty of research has revealed CoQ10's wide range of health benefits.

5. **Take a power nap**. Study after study has shown that a nap of 20-25 minutes is enough to give you an energy boost to make it through the rest of the day.

   Set a timer or the alarm on your mobile phone for the allotted time, and then relax in a quiet place. If your office is too noisy, take a nap in your car. As soon as you feel fatigue washing over you, stop and power nap. You'll be surprisingly alert with just that short period of rest.

Choose several natural energy boosters that will keep you active and alert for many years. Staying fit and healthy and watching after yourself will help Mother Nature provide you with the youthful activity level that you desire.

What to Eat to Live Longer

Eat Brightly coloured fruit and vegetables

A vast amount of well publicised research indicates that those who eat more fruit and vegetables tend to live longer than those who don't, this is due to the nutrients that fruit and veg contain.

There is no doubt that all fruit and veg is good for you, some in plentiful portions and some in moderation but overall the brightly coloured produce is particularly beneficial because the natural pigments which give them their colours can also help prevent cancer.

If ever there was a case history or indeed a race to prove this point it would have to be The Okinawans.

They are reputed to have the world's longest life expectancy and who have low rates of heart disease and cancer. Their diet that is rich in fruit and veg, especially dark green and yellow varieties. In particular, the Okinawan diet features large quantities of sweet potatoes, they replaced the traditional Japanese staple of rice with this vibrant veg.

Okinawa Island is the largest of the Okinawa Islands and the Ryukyu (Nansei) Islands of Japan in the Kyushu region.

You can eat chocolate!

Good news for chocoholics. Cocoa beans are packed with antioxidants and studies have discovered that they can help cut your risk of heart disease.

Don't take this as a license to stock upon chocolate bars, one square a day is enough to boost your health. Make sure you buy the over 70 per cent cocoa bars which contain more flavonoids and less sugar.

Here's an interesting read. https://www.elle.com/beauty/health-fitness/advice/a12666/how-the-chocolate-diet-got-me-healthy/

And more research
https://www.scranton.edu/faculty/vinson/pages/articles-press.shtml

Eat Fish (without the chips)

Which Nation Lives the Longest? – What do they eat?

1. Monaco   89.32 2019 (Est.)

2. Japan   85.77 2019 (Est.)

3. Singapore   85.73 2019 (Est.)

4. Macau   84.6   2019 (Est.)

5. San Marino 83.44 2019 (Est.)

Monaco is top of the list, it is right on the Mediterranean, they eat lots of fresh seafood, olive oil, fruits, vegetables, nuts and whole grains

Japanese people have one of the longest life expectancies in the world, which may be down to their traditional diet this is high in fish.

Singapore is a seaport, they eat lots of fish.

Macau is a hub for many different cuisines because it was governed by Portugal. As well as Cantonese food there is also Portuguese, Japanese, Chinese, and Macanese, seafood plays a pig part in their diet, but Macau street food can be very fatty.

San Marino eat a balance of fruits, vegetables, whole grains, legumes, nuts, fish, and poultry.

Evidence that opting for fish over other meat does reduce your risk of many of the health problems associated with red meat, such as heart disease, but oily fish such as salmon, mackerel, sardines and trout are renowned for their health benefits.

A tin of sardines for example costs a little as 40p and even less in our low-cost supermarkets such as Aldi and Lidl. Both fresh and canned sardines are another healthy option.

Sardines contain far less mercury than most other fish, and a 3.5-ounce serving contains as much omega-3 fatty acids as pink salmon.

Oily fish is a good source of vitamins A and D which are good for the immune system, as well as being rich in omega-3 fatty acids which have been linked to a lowered risk of heart disease, brain damage and stroke.

Scientists have also discovered that the DHA (docosahexaenoic acid) in fish is the key to combating Alzheimer's: DHA slows down the progression of Alzheimer's disease, making this the key ingredient for a healthy brain and, ultimately, a healthier lifestyle too. See link below.

https://www.ncbi.nlm.nih.gov/pubmed/10479465

Green Tea

I mentioned earlier that green tea boasts a vast array of health benefits, it helps to improve cardiovascular health, it regulates our blood pressure, it boosts our immune system, and lowers our cholesterol.

Studies show that drinking green tea, which is rich in health-boosting flavonoids (as is dark chocolate) – can help to lower your risk of cancer.

Coffee!

A study by the University of Scranton found that the flavonoids contained in coffee can prevent heart disease.

https://www.scranton.edu/faculty/vinson/pages/articles-press.shtml#6

Dr. Joe Vinson, the professor who led the research, says that "antioxidants are your army to protect you from the toxic free radicals, which come from breathing oxygen and eating sugar, that start chronic diseases".

The antioxidants in coffee ward off life-threatening diseases such as cancer, heart disease, diabetes, and stroke.

So, before you start quaffing coffee by the mug load, be mindful, that caffeine raises our blood pressure, thus a large amount of coffee isn't good and it's best to opt for decaf, which offers the same amount of antioxidant properties as regular coffee.

Olive Oil versus Rapeseed Oil

Oil in our food has always been a bone of contention and indeed many of us give fats and oils a wide berth in a bid to stay trim and healthy.

We shouldn't ignore the 'good' monounsaturated fats, which are found in olive oil, are claimed to be essential for good health. There has been many studies findings that regular consumption of olive oil can help cut the risk of stroke and heart disease, due to its high content of micronutrients called phenols which have anti-inflammatory and antioxidant properties.

We are all aware that olive oil a staple of Mediterranean diet and linking it with longevity.

What of the new kid on the block… rapeseed oil?

Is rapeseed oil a healthier alternative to our trusty olive oil?.

In fairness we need to compare olive oil with rapeseed oil so we can understand who the winner in the healthy oil stakes is.

Olive oil has a long history and is well known for its protective properties in maintaining a healthy heart, with the virgin olive oils containing an even wider range of antioxidant plant compounds and vitamin E.

The main type of fat in olive oil is monounsaturated which helps prevent cholesterol being deposited on artery walls and therefore helps to protect us from cardiovascular disease.

We have seen the fancy labels telling us 'early pressings of the olives' on extra virgin olive oil bottles, as well as 'cold pressed' oil produce.

This is an olive oil that is rich in beneficial plant compounds. These polyphenols can protect against cancer, high blood pressure, lower cholesterol and the compound oleocanthal, an anti- inflammatory with similar action to ibuprofen.

Olive oil like rapeseed oil is rich in antioxidant vitamin E.

Be careful how you store your olive oil as researchers in Italy have found that light destroys many of the disease – fighting compounds in olive oil so be careful how you store it. The lovely expensive bottle of your kitchen windowsill may not be the best place!

Studies have also showed that after a year, the olive oil stored in clear bottles under store lighting showed at least 30% decrease in antioxidants.

There are some after-purchase ground rules with olive oil, such as being stored in the dark and used within one to two months.

Also, to enjoy the full benefit of olive oil, eat it cold. Don't use extra virgin olive oil for cooking at high temperatures because the beneficial chemicals will be destroyed.

The case for rapeseed oil.

Rapeseed oil is certainly one of the healthiest oils.

It is nearly as high in monounsaturated fat as olive oil and contains much higher amounts of omega-3 fat.

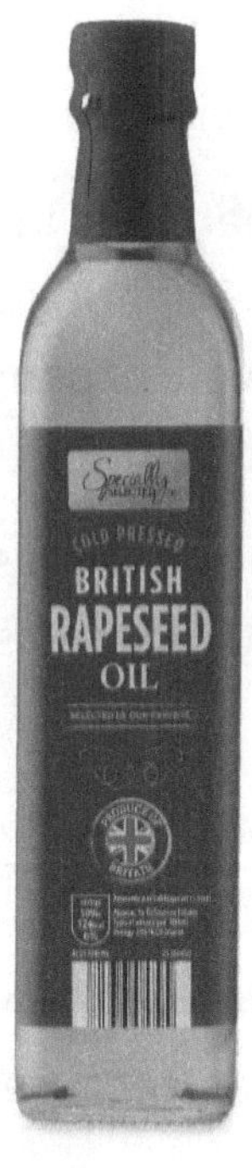

Rapeseed oil has a host of health benefits when eaten regularly, more so than in any other oil used in quantity for culinary purposes.

Rapeseed oil has a perfect balance between omega-6 and omega-3s and is lower in saturated fat than all commonly used oils.

Rapeseed oil contains no artificial preservatives and is trans-fat and GM free. It is suitable for a variety of diets – vegetarian, gluten-free, Kosher and Halal.

Rapeseed oil is safe to cook with at high temperatures, it has a burning point of 230 ºC much higher than olive oil which typically ranges from 185ºC- 204 ºC depending on the variety of oil.

Both olive oil and rapeseed oil are good choices as they are high in unsaturated fatty acids. However, rapeseed oil has less unhealthy saturated fat than most cooking oils – 50% less than olive oil and a fraction of that of palm oil.

So, in this olive oil vs rapeseed oil focus, rapeseed oil in many ways has an even better 'health profile' than olive oil does, Rapeseed oil contains an excellent balance of essential fats in line with recommended guidelines.

Refined rapeseed oil is a good choice for cooking because it doesn't degrade when heated.

Cold pressed or extra virgin rapeseed oil is great choice for salad dressings and drizzling.

Thanks to North Norfolk Nutrition

What about the price of olive oil and rapeseed oil?

500 ml Cold pressed Rapeseed oil at Aldi £1.49
500 ml Extra Virgin Olive Oil at Aldi £2.59

500 ml Cold pressed Rapeseed oil at Waitrose £4.80
500 ml Extra Virgin Olive Oil at Waitrose £2.15

500 ml Cold pressed Rapeseed oil at Tesco £3.00
500 ml Extra Virgin Olive Oil at Tesco £3.25

Let's have a look at the labels on both olive oil and rapeseed oil.

Olive oil per 1 tablespoon/15ml serving	Cold pressed Rapeseed oil per 1tablespoon/15ml serving
Kcal 123	Kcal 124
Protein 0g	Protein 0g
Carbohydrate 0g	Carbohydrate 0g
Sugar 0g	Sugar 0g
Total fat 13.7g	Total Fat 13.1g
Saturated fat 2.1g	Saturated fat 1g
Monounsaturated fat 10.01g	Monounsaturated 8.0g
Polyunsaturated 1.13g	Polyunsaturated 4.2g
Sodium 0 mg	Sodium 0 mg

Cranberries

Cranberries, not too long ago seemed to only appear in a jelly to help make our dried-up Christmas turkey tastes better but as time has moved on cranberries offer many health benefits, but, can it be classed as a 'life-saver'?

Well the cranberry is full of antioxidants, anti-inflammatory, antibacterial and immune-boosting properties, as well as being jam-packed full of phytonutrients. The more phytonutrients we have in our body, the greater the protection we have.

The phytochemicals found in red fruits and berries help to combat cancer-causing molecules.

In a study conducted by Cornell University, researchers tested cranberry extracts on human breast cancer cells and discovered that, over four hours, many of the same breast cancer cells had begun to die.

https://www.ncbi.nlm.nih.gov/pubmed/16377076

Garlic

Garlic as always been one of the good guys, except when it's on someone's breath but a vast amount of evidence tells us that of the many compounds found in garlic, 10 of them help to combat cancer.

https://www.aicr.org/foods-that-fight-cancer/garlic.html

Garlic contains immune-enhancing compounds that help to break down the substances that cause cancer.

For example, diallyl sulphide is a component of garlic and is known for its ability to break down carcinogens in the body, which may have led to cancer if they weren't destroyed.

According to research, people who consume garlic regularly face half the risk of stomach cancer than those who eat little or none.

Summary

So, we do have the power to change many of the variables that influence how long we live, and how active and vital we feel in our later years.

There are actions that we can take to increase our odds of a longer and more satisfying life span.

Here's the top ten of the many and various actions we can take to help us live longer:

1. Quit smoking.
2. Do some physical and mental activities every day.
3. Eat a healthy diet rich in whole grains, vegetables, and fruits, and substitute healthier monounsaturated and polyunsaturated fats for unhealthy saturated fats and trans fats.
4. Consider taking a daily multivitamin, and be sure to get enough calcium and vitamin D.
5. Maintain a healthy weight and body shape.
6. Challenge your brain. Keep learning and trying new activities.
7. Build a strong social network.
8. Follow preventive care and screening guidelines.
9. Floss, brush, and see a dentist regularly.

10. last but by no means least, ask your doctor if there are medications that can help you control the potential long-term side effects of chronic conditions such as high blood pressure, osteoporosis, or high cholesterol.